In the Hands of Her Caregivers

by

Marilyn Mitchell

In the Hands of Her Caregivers

Marilyn Mitchell © 2022

Cover design by Aknowingspirit LLC

ISBN: 978-1-7377860-1-6

Ordering Information:

Quantity sales. Special discounts are available on quantity purchases by churches, associations, and others. For details, contact the author at the address below. Orders by trade bookstores and wholesalers. Please email admin@aknowingspirit.com.

Dedication

To mummy, in loving memory.

To the Dr. Jimmys of the world.

To Aunt Merle Collins for the tremendous love and support you provided in helping to put my thoughts together for this book.

To my many aunts, you know who you are, father, grandmother, uncles, cousins and many friends who have been very supportive.

Also to my husband who came to my life after the first draft was written and has always been a big support.

Chapter 1

"Are you going to call it?"

"No. I have a faint pulse, let's keep going."

When she woke up and could talk to them again, she told them that story. Although the conversation seemed far away, she could hear them deciding. Denise wanted to know who the nurse was that ended up helping her to live.

But that was later. Before and after that moment, much had happened.

***

Emergency room

"Ouch!" Denise uttered that sound as an intense pain shot through her back. It was sudden and very different from the pain she had experienced before. This scared her. Trembling, she decided to take the advice of her physicians, family, and friends and go to the emergency room at Northern Metropolitan Hospital.

The hospital is in a downtown neighborhood in Montgomery County, Maryland. Northern Metropolitan is a community-based hospital, known as a trauma center.

It was the day after Thanksgiving 2016 and Denise had been experiencing back pain but had little relief from the Tylenol and Tramadol prescribed to her. For the last ten days, she had been taking them daily. Denise would often joke about having an elevated level of tolerance for pain. For days, she tried to manage on her own the rapidly intensifying aches. She took the medication prescribed religiously, hoping for relief. After ignoring the pain for so long, Denise finally relented and spoke to her daughter Mara and close friend Breana.

"Mummy, I'm worried." Mara said, unable to mask the anxiety building inside her. Breana's concern was expressed differently. She immediately started with questions.

"What is this pain about? How long has this been happening?" she said, not mincing her words. "This must be why I'm having pain."

.   Denise, attempting to quell their concerns, reminded them about her medical history of hypertension, gastroesophageal reflux disease (GERD), aortic dissection, abdominal aneurysm, and stroke.

"This must be why I'm having pain." She spoke.

While Mara and Breana agreed, they encouraged her to find the exact cause and reason for the intense pain.

At 61 years old, Denise enjoyed spending time with her family, friends, and colleagues. She was full of life, and especially loved to travel. Denise enjoyed annual trips to Grenada, West Indies to visit her mother, siblings, relatives and childhood friends. In fact, she and Mara, had gone to visit her mother two months earlier to celebrate her mother's birthday.

Denise had survived an aortic dissection six years prior and was back to her baseline. She did not use any assistive devices, she was independent with activities of daily living, worked full time in an office setting, and managed her own home, except for one thing: She could not drive.

"Mummy, I cannot be driving you around all the time. You must get your license." Mara said, jokingly but serious.

Denise, with a beatific smile, shrugged helplessly, barely hiding her round dimpled face and laughing eyes.

"Well, Mara ..."

Mara understood that statement. It meant her mother had a deep fear of negotiating traffic, and because of that, there was not an ounce of regret or even guilt about not having her driver's license. Besides, this was their time to bond. The front passenger's seat of Mara's car became her mother's rightful place. In truth, Mara did not mind. Denise was a great navigator, trip planner, and companion. Nevertheless, Mara had to drop hints about the driver's license, just in case Denise changed her mind.

But this time was not a casual trip to the store. It was a trip to the emergency room and Mara was not with her. Denise was afraid. She took a cab to the emergency room. As she sat in the emergency waiting room, the thought of an aortic dissection weighed heavily on her mind. Her experience with the long emergency room wait was no different from any other time that she had spent in the emergency room. Her complaints were not perceived as a true emergency by the emergency room personnel. Denise waited for hours before a nurse or doctor dealt with her.

As she waited, she maintained contact with Mara, via text messages.

Denise: *At Northern Metropolitan Hospital, registered and waiting to be seen. The nurse does not believe I am dissecting. It happens faster.*

Mara: *You still need a CT scan or MRI to see what's happening.*

Denise : *Yes*

An hour and a half go by.

Mara: *Is it busy? Hopefully, I will hear something soon. I just called you.*

Five minutes later, another text from Mara.

Are you ok?

Still no response. Mara wondered what was going on, but she was not worried because she assumed that her mother was undergoing tests in the emergency room. She waited three hours. Then she called the emergency room to enquire about Denise's status.

"Your mom is okay." The nurse said. "She's in a room here in the emergency room. She is stable. Perhaps her phone battery died. I will tell her that you called."

Approximately fifteen minutes later, Denise called. "I am okay. They were doing tests so I could not use the phone. Then they were trying to put an IV line and they were having a tough time finding a vein, but they finally got one."

All afternoon, between texting Mara and waiting to be seen, Denise could only think of her experiences with aortic dissection and prayed it wasn't that.

Chapter 2

Aortic dissection 2010: "What's wrong with my heart?"

It had happened in January, six years before. Most of what Denise knew about it was what family and friends had told her, but there were a few key factors that she remembered.

In January 2010, she had been out of work for about a week, suffering from what she thought was a cold. To get clearance to return to work, she went to the neighborhood clinic, as her primary care physician was out of town. Prior to going to the clinic, she medicated herself with over-the-counter cold remedies. Denise realized that given her history of hypertension, she had taken too much of them. The realization came when she started a second bottle of cold medicine. Eventually, Denise was discharged from the clinic with a prescription and with Mara she drove to the nearby pharmacy, dropped off the prescription and were told to wait approximately 40 minutes.

They decided to walk across the parking lot to a store where Denise wanted to look at lamps. As they reached the back of the store, Mara noticed the visible change in her mom.

"Mummy, your whole face just took on a different expression. I was scared." Mara said, continuing to scan her face for more signs of pain. Without warning, Denise cried out, clasping her hands at the center of her jacket. "Oh God! My chest... My back! Mara! My chest, my chest!"

Her mother's breathing was rapid and labored and it was clear this was an emergency. Mara guided Denise to a chair nearby.

"My blood pressure was high in the clinic." Denise whispered trying to catch her breath. Mara immediately called 911, then called her brother Malcolm. It was not long before customers began to gather and assist. "It will be okay." A lady said using a fan to keep her cool. Mara could tell her mom needed reassurance.

Within a few minutes, paramedics arrived. They took her vitals which showed a blood pressure reading of 206/125. Mara held her jacket, bag, and phone while the medics continued to assess her. Her cell phone rang. It was the clinic.

"Ms. Mitchell, you forgot to pick up the return-to-work note. Would you be able to come back to pick it up? It will be at the front desk."

***

Denise reflected on that moment, and even as she sat in the waiting room now, anxious about everything, she had to smile to herself. She remembered Mara responding to the call from the pharmacy in that tight little voice, "I just called 911 for my mother. Her blood pressure is extremely high." That was all.

Denise did not know why, of all things, she remembered that moment so clearly. Sometimes she would look her at daughter—body still so small and slim, and wonder if she was really a big person? But when she was annoyed, there was no question. When Mara is upset she lets you know it. The thought of Mara brought a smile to Denise's face.

The rest of the story Denise only knows from what they told her afterwards—what Mara told her, and what other people filled in from having heard some of it from Mara. The paramedics told them that they were taking Denise to the nearest hospital, the St. John's Hospital, and that she should meet them there. And she half-remembered other things that Mara said later.

"Mummy, you started to give orders, telling me who to call, 'Mara call Myrna. Call Malcolm, Breana, Lori, Cathy. Call Jenice. Tell them I am going to the hospital."

She began giving those instructions even while complaining of the excruciating pain. And she kept crying, "Oh my God, my children." And even then,

Mara's sense of humor was trying to put things in perspective. Denise said later to her friend Myrna, "Mara not easy, you hear! She said she was just hoping that no one would ask her how old these children were." And Denise reflected when she told the story later, both are adults, it is true, not of the age when they would be eager to share that information with strangers. But ... well, your children are your children." And she usually ended her recounting with "They brought me out to the ambulance and ... Mara really knows the rest of the story."

Diagnostics at Northern Metropolitan Hospital

"Ms. Mitchell, you're going to radiology for a CT scan now," her nurse said peeking through the curtain. She pulled the curtain open and a tall, slender, young woman with blonde shoulder length hair was standing next to the nurse.

"Hi, I'm Kyle." She said to Denise with a bright comforting smile.

"Hi Kyle..." Denise replied.

Wasting no time, Kyle walked over to the stretcher, and released the brakes, "Okay, off we go!"

Mara's Version: 2010 Cross-State Journey to the Hospital

Mara always goes back in her thoughts to 2010 and the events leading up to and after the aortic dissection. She remembers the ambulance. The crew brought her mother out to the ambulance and took a few minutes before they started to drive. She remembers waiting, wondering why it was taking them so long to drive off when they had an emergency. When the ambulance drove off, she drove off. She could not help wondering why the ambulance was moving so slowly. Was this how they always did things?

The ambulance drove without lights and sirens. That was even more worrisome. She had expected them to drive full speed, with lights and sirens—signaling an emergency. Eventually, the ambulance got there, with Mara's car following closely. The ambulance drove straight ahead toward the emergency room entrance and Mara followed the signs for patients' and visitors' parking. She was incredibly nervous, thinking about her mother and every space was too small for her car.

She drove around a bit in the parking lot, until she came back to the first space that she had seen. She parked, walked toward the emergency room entrance, and found the front desk.

"Hello, my mother, Denise Mitchell just came in."

"Hi, please take a seat and they'll call you when you can go back to see her." The attendant responded.

Mara sat in the waiting room for half an hour. Then the attendant called her to the desk, "Ms. Mitchell, you can go in to see your mom. "She's in 1A."

Mara walked through the door that the attendant opened for her and walked toward 1A. She saw her mother. Denise was slouched on a stretcher in what Mara concluded from her mother's expression was obvious pain. She looked at the monitor and saw that her mother's blood pressure was now just as high as it had been when the paramedics took the vital signs at the store.

"Did they give you anything for pain?" Mara said trying to piece together what had happened in her absence.

Denise lifted her head to look at her daughter. Her eyes were red, as though she had been crying.

"No, they didn't give me anything."

Mara immediately looked up and called for the first nurse she saw walking by.

"Excuse me, can she get something for pain?"

"Um, let me check the orders."

The nurse stopped in front of the stretcher, then continued in the direction of the nursing station. Mara tried to console her mother who was groaning.

"You'll be okay mummy, try to sit back."

"No, I can't." Her mother said showing signs of discomfort.

Twenty minutes later, Malcolm arrived. He sat on the chair next to Mara, who updated him about the events leading up to that point, including the request for pain medication for their mother, that still had not arrived. Shortly after that, Mara's friend Pria joined them. Pria usually worked there in the emergency room, but it was her day off. It was good to see her. Mara felt this was someone who knew the space, and could help.

St. John's Hospital

They sat near their mother in the emergency room and watched her. Denise was clearly uncomfortable on the stretcher. She was unable to sit back as the back pain was more excruciating in that position. It was difficult for Mara to watch her mother writhe in pain, unable to help in any way. She could see that it was hard for Malcolm, too.

The nurse assigned to Denise walked by a couple of times, and Mara and Malcolm asked her again for their mother to be medicated. Mara tried not to be impatient. This was her profession, too. She was in the health field. She reminded herself that the physician was trying to determine the diagnosis before medicating her mother. Still, she felt helpless. Mara asked another nurse walking by to make her mother comfortable. Something had to be done by the staff.

On behalf of her mother, Mara made a few phone calls to notify family and friends. She knew that within a few minutes an informal phone tree would form, and soon everyone whom her mother wanted to be notified would be notified. The message would also be sent to individuals that Denise had not mentioned, including those whom Mara did not know.

Mara was particularly anxious to speak with Auntie Breana, her mother's close friend. Breana was not only a close friend but also a nurse with over twenty-five years of experience. She was a nursing director at another hospital and Mara knew that in this situation she would be a great resource. On the phone, Mara kept Auntie Breana updated regarding Denise's vital signs. Mara also phoned and maintained contact with her friend Miranda, also a nurse, who gave her opinions and support. Having so many friends in the health field was reassuring and it helped—but it still was not easy to watch her mother's discomfort while they waited for a diagnosis.

Diagnosis

Denise was diagnosed by the physician in the emergency room with a thoracic aortic dissection in the ascending aorta. She required surgery and needed to be medivacked to a tertiary care hospital. Malcolm and Mara were approached by one of the doctors in the emergency room. He presented them with two options for possible transfer—of course, the decision would also be based on bed availability and an accepting physician at the other hospital.

Later, when Denise learned that her son had selected the University Hospital, she was grateful. The helicopter transported Denise. The siblings and their friend drove to the University Hospital, which was approximately 50 minutes away, or it would be fifty minutes under normal circumstances. On this occasion, the three climbed into Mara's car. Mara sat in the back seat, Pria took the front passenger's seat and Malcolm sat in the driver's seat. He drove because he was more familiar with the area where the University Hospital was located. As one might expect under the circumstances, their drive took 35 minutes.

University Hospital

When they arrived at the hospital, Denise was being admitted by the nurse to the cardiac intensive care unit. The staff allowed them in to visit soon after they arrived. Their friend Pria prayed at the bedside. When Denise woke up three hours later, she did not know where she was and was surprised to hear that she was at a hospital that was an hour away from her house. She was also surprised to learn that she had been transported via a helicopter. She had been vomiting in the emergency room at the previous hospital and was administered pain and nausea medications by the nurse. She had fallen asleep soon after she was medicated and woke up at a different hospital. Denise tried to act calm, but it was obvious to Mara that she was scared. The anesthesiologist explained his role in her care, and Denise was alert enough to question him.

"I'm relying on you to remember that you need to wake me up after the procedure." She informed him.

He smiled, confirming that he understood the task. Mara could see her mother's eyes crinkle in an attempt at the usual ever-ready smile. Denise took a good look at the anesthesiologist.

"You seem so young." She said. "I just want to make sure that you're capable of doing the job."

He could not help but laugh. Mara knew that her mother was afraid of having surgery, nonetheless she was very much there, though. Humor, Mara felt, was her way of both coping and letting them know that she wanted to be involved in her care. It was her usual way. Her mother wanted to be sure that those at the facility knew she was a human being. Her mother's banter was reassuring. It was much needed confirmation that she was alive and alert.

Pre-operative

Dr. Jimmy, the surgeon, was called in by his department from home. He arrived and met Denise's children in the consultation room. Mara should've dressed appropriately for outdoors before leaving the house, but thought she was just going to the walk-in clinic a few minutes away from her mother's house. The consultation room was very cold. Mara and Malcolm were given blankets by the nurses in order to turn the sofas into makeshift beds. She tried to make herself comfortable. Mara removed her shoes and hoped the jeans and the sweater she wore would be enough to keep her warm. Unfortunately, her socks were not much help. There was a noticeable hole in one side—exposing her toe.

Dr. Jimmy, explained their mother's condition, and would often stare toward the floor for several minutes as he spoke.

"Is he looking at the hole in my sock?" Mara wondered, growing uncomfortable at the thought. She kept adjusting to hide the hole, convinced that Dr. Jimmy was probably distracted by the sight. Mara masked her embarrassment and focused on what Dr. Jimmy was saying.

"Your mother is in very critical condition." He said plainly. "And that procedure is very risky."

Dr. Jimmy went on to explain that her blood pressure was so elevated that the pressure made a tear through the aorta—the largest artery in the body that carries blood away from the heart to the rest of the body.

"Do everything you can to bring my mother back." Mara said, completely forgetting about how she may have been perceived hole in sock and all.

Mara was unsure if her words made an impact, regardless, there was no denying Dr. Jimmy did a remarkable job. Throughout the ordeal, the staff was hospitable. They allowed the family to use the consultation room as their own private space. After that day, while Denise remained at the hospital, that room became Mara's sleeping quarters.

Post-operative care

In the early morning hours, Denise was taken by the surgical team to surgery. Her heart stopped three times after the procedure and the staff, having been told that her daughter Mara was a recovery room nurse, provided updates to her as if this were one of her patients. They told her to face the possibility that her mother would not survive. Mara sobbed in her aunt Myrna's arms. It was approaching 12:30 in the afternoon when that most upsetting update came from the nurse liaison who updated families.

Remarkably, later, Denise told her family and friends that she heard someone say, "It's 12:28, are you going to call it?" She also recalled hearing another voice answer, "No I have a faint pulse, let's keep going." She also remembered seeing her younger brother Reynold, who was deceased, telling her to stay because her children needed her. But all that information came later.

Now, while they waited, the nurse returned to the consultation room to update Mara, Myrna, and Malcolm's ex-girlfriend, that Denise had regained a pulse. Mara reflected later that it was while Denise was traveling to that other place and meeting deceased relatives, that she asked the liaison if she could see her mother. At the time her heart stopped, Denise was in her room in the cardiac intensive care unit. She had been transported by the surgical team back to her room on that floor, from the operating room, to allow her body temperature to stabilize. Her temperature was exceptionally low in the operating room. The surgical team's plan was to take her back to the operating room when she was stable. Her chest was open. The liaison told Mara that she would be able to have a glimpse of her mother in the hallway, as they wheeled her back to the operating room.

The liaison was a Caucasian woman about five feet three inches tall. She had short blonde hair. She had a round face with rosy cheeks. She wore light blue scrubs with a white lab coat over the scrubs. She sat down next to Mara. Looking directly into her eyes and turning her blue eyes from side to side to include everyone, the liaison explained that the physician assistant would be massaging Denise's heart as they transported her, so they would be moving quickly, and Denise would not be exposed. It happened as she was told by the liaison.

As Mara stood in the hallway, the staff moved briskly as they transported Denise, but she could see the physician assistant's hand underneath the sheet. He acknowledged Denise's family standing in the hallway with a nod and the group kept moving swiftly.

As the news spread of Denise's condition and admission to the University hospital, family and friends arrived at the hospital to show their support. It seemed like an eternity as they waited until Denise returned from the operating room and was allowed to have visitors. They congregated in the consultation room.

"Our father, who art in heaven..." they prayed aloud as a group. Some of them were meeting for the first time and others reconnected.
"Myrna, I did not know you were here. I thought I heard you had gone back to Grenada."
"James, good to see you. Long time. Not nice circumstances, but still..."

Mara could not help thinking that, lying ill on her hospital bed, her mother was doing what she always did: bringing people together.

Denise spent approximately nine days on the ventilator. She recovered.

"Denise suffered a stroke during the procedure." The surgeon explained. "Some calcium escaped into her brain and the left side of her body was affected."

Mara did not immediately react, she just listened. Mara thought there was no blame to be ascribed for this mishap. She still thought the team was wonderful. Their attitude alone said they were committed to their patient. To her, it was inspiring to see the way they worked and interacted with the family. The physician assistant also met with a consultation room filled with family and friends and updated them on her status. He answered questions with Mara's permission as it was her mother's medical information being shared. Denise and everyone connected to her was happy that she survived.

***

Mara sent out a hundred text messages to update family and friends. She asked for prayers because the family agreed, Denise needed prayers. The healthcare providers who cared for her mother did everything that they could, but family and friends felt there was a higher power who was responsible.

Her mother's close friend Ali contacted the Catholic church and requested that the priest visit Denise.

Later, Denise told family and friends that when she woke up on the ventilator, she thought that someone had kidnapped her. Staff wore masks and gowns and it all looked strange when she woke up in the cardiac intensive care unit. She could not see the faces of these figures covered with caps and gowns. She could not move her head. All she could see was that they approached her with syringes and moved their hands toward her, attending, she later discovered, to an intravenous line on her neck. They spoke but because of the masks, she was unable to hear or understand what they said. She saw Mara, and all she could think was, 'they got you too?' She wondered where she and her daughter had been found and kidnapped, and what exactly was happening. When Mara heard her mother's story later, she thought what a good thing it was that she had spoken to her mother when she saw that she had opened her eyes. She spoke to her mother reassuringly, told her that she was okay and explained to her what had happened. The explanation was what brought her mother back to an awareness of her surroundings.

While Denise remained on the ventilator on the cardiac intensive care unit, the physical and occupational therapists provided therapy. They could only do limited exercise, but they were able to get some done at the bedside.

Later, in the intermediate care unit, after the medical team weaned her off the ventilator, Denise spoke with what her daughter Mara thought was a British accent. When the multidisciplinary team walked in the hallway on the unit as they discussed their patients' plan of care, otherwise known as rounding, they stopped in front of Denise's room. She saw them through the glass doors from her room. She waved at them and said, "Hello, hello" with her British accent. Mara almost giggled, wondering what was happening. It seemed odd to her that this was her mother's new way of communicating after her experience. Wherever she had traveled to, she had come back with a British accent. Was this a journey back to her British colonial education? Was she getting an accent from the voices in her books? Was this from the British comedy programs she liked? Of course, the British speech was short-lived, for about a few days.

Her friends and family were astonished by her accent but were extremely happy and thankful to hear her voice and to have her back. Mara reflected that her mother had always enjoyed British shows, comedy as well as drama. She somehow must have been able to relate to the characters or the world in which those characters lived after her near-death experience. Watching her mother, Mara marveled at the workings of the human mind.

On the intermediate care unit, Denise received more physical and occupational therapy services. She walked in the hallway with the therapists, with a walker. She smiled proudly as her visitors cheered her on. She needed to take several short breaks and the therapists were very patient and allowed her sufficient time during their sessions.

***

Acute rehabilitation hospital

After three and a half weeks, on February 16th, 2010, the University Hospital transferred Denise to an acute rehabilitation hospital in Washington DC, where she received superb care that allowed her to have a full recovery. The therapists were aware that she had been independent prior to her hospitalization. They knew that she had suffered a stroke during the procedure for the aortic dissection and recognized her motivation to recover fully. They collaborated with her to help achieve her goals. Looking back to 2010 from new experiences of the system in 2016, Mara thinks that these were good memories of the hospital and health care system.

Later, after she recovered and was at home with family, Denise commended the therapists for their commitment and encouragement for her full recovery. She spoke about the occupational therapist who went into the shower with her to ensure that she cleaned herself thoroughly and to ensure her safety. She recalled how she sobbed and how embarrassed she felt that she needed help to shower and how the therapist reassured her that she would be able to independently care for herself in time. She acknowledged the patience and kindness that the therapists gave not just to her but to other patients whom she met in the group activities. Her daughter attended four of her therapy sessions and Denise seemed happy. Involvement of family and friends, Mara reflected, can help with the recovery process. Subsequent experiences made her think about this and reflect that healthcare providers should not treat such involvement as an interference to the delivery of care.

Discharge planning

As Denise approached her discharge date from the acute rehabilitation hospital popularly known as acute rehab, the rehab team held a discharge planning meeting. These facilities, get mixed reviews throughout the country. On this occasion, Denise's experience was a positive one.

The discharge planner was very professional. She explained the discharge process. She informed Denise and Mara that she had ordered durable medical equipment such as a rolling walker, an elevated toilet seat and a tub bench to be delivered by the equipment company to Denise's home address. The physical and occupational therapists made the recommendations for the durable medical equipment. If the health insurance company would cover payment for the equipment, the discharge planner would proceed with ordering the equipment with a doctor's order. The discharge planner also explained that Denise would benefit from outpatient therapy for a while and so she had arranged the services with an outpatient facility near Denise's residence. She suggested that Denise would qualify for Metro Access, a shared ride service that would transport her to and from appointments and the discharge planner helped Denise and Mara to initiate the application process. She provided them with supplies for dressing changes for Denise's incision and gave Mara information on how to order additional supplies.

Much was dependent not only on the services provided by the facility, but also on Denise's health insurance and the services that would be considered appropriate.

Mara's knowledge of the health care system helped here. She had some sense of what was legally due her mother and what the insurance services might provide.

Discharge from acute rehab

After spending a little less than two weeks at the acute rehab, the physician discharged Denise to her home on February 27th, 2010, with an open incision. Inside her home, there were about twelve steps from the ground floor, where the kitchen, dining and living area were, up to the bedroom and three steps to the exterior of the house. Denise was able to maneuver her way up and down these steps because the therapists had worked well with her, both at the University Hospital and at the acute rehabilitation hospital. At first, she avoided climbing up and down the stairs for four weeks, except when she was going to outpatient therapy. She confined herself to her bedroom and was content with receiving room service. Mara functioned as her home care nurse, packing the incision daily, following the doctor's orders and discharge instructions received from the acute rehab.

One of Denise's sisters, Yvonne, traveled from Grenada to stay at home with her for five weeks. Yvonne took time-off from her job to be able to help Denise, who appreciated the support. Another sister, Simone, also traveled from Grenada. Simone was a physician, and her involvement in Denise's recovery was extremely helpful. Other friends and relatives contributed in other ways. It was an all-hands on deck approach in Denise's recovery, which meant that one or two individuals would not feel overwhelmed with providing support to Denise. The equipment that the discharge planner ordered arrived at the house. Metro Access transported her back and forth to her outpatient therapy on the days that Mara was not available to transport her. She barely used the walker, as she was determined to be back to her baseline.

Approximately six months after she was discharged from the acute care rehab, when she felt physically able to return to her paying job, Denise continued to be transported to work with the shared ride services by Metro Access. Initially, she was on a half day schedule at the office, until she eventually worked her full eight-hour schedule. Denise was back to her baseline within a year, with no residual effects from the stroke.

Back to her baseline: and at work

Denise worked at an international financial organization in Washington D.C. and required occasional travel abroad. Her last trip overseas for work was one to Europe. She enjoyed traveling, and there were upcoming trips that she hoped to be a part of—including one to West Africa.

Denise's role involved attending and making preparations for conferences. A year after the aortic dissection, the physicians recommended that she refrain from taking long-distance flights or visiting places where it may be difficult to return to the United States in the event of a medical emergency. Although disappointed, she followed their advice. Adjustments were made to her job requirements to include no travel abroad. Again, a great disappointment, but Denise understood.

Chapter 3

Survivors of aortic dissection

Denise resumed usual activities after being discharged from the acute rehab. However, there were moments of concern. There were two incidents of temporary blindness, when she woke up unable to see. They were the first notable symptomatic occurrences after exposure to heparin.

The first incident occurred approximately eight months after her discharge from the acute rehab and the second was in November 2010, a month after the first incident. She was hospitalized in Washington D.C. after the second event, but a neurology check did not reveal anything. Her cardiologist told her that the temporary blindness was due to a delayed reaction from heparin, an anticoagulant that is used to prevent blood clots. It was unclear how much of that information the providers documented in the records of the various institutions, but Denise communicated this to all her providers. Approximately one year after the physician discharged her from the acute rehab, on February 28th, 2011, she complained of abdominal pain to her cardiologist—who then ordered a CT scan. The CT scan indicated that she had an abdominal aneurysm which is an enlargement of the aorta, the main blood vessel that delivers blood to the body, at the level of the abdomen. Her cardiologist told her that she would not need to have surgery to repair it because it was not large enough to require surgery. Whenever she experienced any chest, abdominal or back pain, her complaints were taken seriously by her doctors, family, and friends, given her history of an aortic dissection. That significant aspect of her medical history was considered by those who took medicine or health seriously, and by members of her family and friend circle knowledgeable enough to recognize the signs and realize the dangers.

On October 7th, 2011, at the hospital where her cardiologist worked, Denise and her daughter waited in the emergency room from 7pm until 4am. Eventually, an emergency room doctor dealt with her and discharged her to home without a diagnosis. Then on May 12th, 2012, she visited the emergency room at the hospital close to her house, again with complaints of abdominal pain. At that time, the doctors admitted her the facility. The emergency room doctor diagnosed bowel obstruction.

As Denise went through these visits to various doctors and hospitals, she was often uneasy.

She was not convinced about the expertise of some of the medical personnel and she always thought about Dr. Jimmy at the University Hospital. Her experience there had been so positive that she thought he would be able to address her health issues, no matter what they were. He was her hero. She thought of him as a concerned, approachable medical practitioner, and she wished she could talk to him. She had almost died, and he had saved her life. He had done it with style, she thought. He showed concern. He was self-confident and he had given her confidence. She researched his accomplishments and kept herself informed about his works. She also researched support groups for survivors of aortic dissection. She read about other individuals' stories and was surprised to discover many others with experiences like hers. She was not only pleased with the surgeon but with the entire multidisciplinary team that had been involved in her care and saved her life. After that episode, she regularly saw a cardiologist to whom one of her friends had referred her. She quoted a phrase from him to her daughter, "You can't be so afraid to die that you stop living." Apart from dealing with everyday stressors in life, she lived. About two years after the aortic dissection, she began to travel abroad, mostly to Grenada to visit her family.

And so, as Denise sat in the emergency room at the Northern Metropolitan Hospital on that day after Thanksgiving 2016, her mind drifted to all the events of 2010 and subsequent years.

Chapter 4

Admit to ICU

On November 25, 2016, Denise spent approximately nine hours in the emergency room at the Northern Metropolitan Hospital. Mara walked in while Denise's nurse returned to her bedside.

Mara realized that the two were continuing a conversation about retirement that must have started before her arrival. As she watched her mother on the stretcher, she realized by her occasional grimaces that Denise was still experiencing back pain. She wondered if her mother's high tolerance for pain explained the nurse's opinion that it could not be an aortic dissection. After spending the entire day in the emergency room, Denise was transferred to a room on the critical care unit to be monitored closely.

She completed an Advance Directive, a written statement about her wishes regarding medical treatment in the event she was unable to communicate them to her doctor. She designated Mara as the primary agent on the Advance

Directive, which meant that Mara would make decisions on her behalf. A couple of days passed with Denise in critical care but her doctor at the hospital did not provide her with a diagnosis. The nursing staff performed bedside report —the outgoing nurse would provide a report to the oncoming nurse. Denise was not a shy patient. She always participated. She described her symptoms to the nurses. Some nurses appreciated their patient's input, some did not. Some, Mara thought, were quite nice and others focused on their tasks and were uninterested in the patient's comments. The bedside reports were helpful as they allowed patients and their families to be involved in their care and to be apprised of the plan of care. It was also time-consuming, as some patients such as Denise enjoyed participating and time did not always afford engagement with every patient during their report. Mara reflected that the facility was more focused on the business aspects of the interaction than on care. She thought that this is happening increasingly in care facilities. People have less time. The business model is taking over.

While on the unit, per the doctor's order, the nurses kept Denise on bedrest with bathroom privileges. The staff limited her activities, to help to control her high blood pressure. On one occasion, she had an episode of dizziness and lightheadedness while she was out of bed to go to the bathroom. After that incident, the nurses instructed her to call for assistance whenever she needed to go to the bathroom.

The staff allowed Denise to have visitors, and she was pleased because she was a very sociable person. Several of her friends, including those from her job, were eager to see her and vice versa. Nichelle, her close friend, and her son visited, and they spoke about her family and the job. Four of Mara's friends also visited. Her friend Miranda visited with her father, who prayed at the bedside for Denise's healing, as he had a strong Christian faith. Miranda is a nurse practitioner and her nursing background helped. She is of Jamaican descent, brown in complexion. She has a quiet demeanor except when the topic is related to nursing issues. She voices her opinions, always in a professional manner. She would always walk directly up to a person, maintaining at least six feet in distance and speak with confidence. She makes eye contact when she speaks and gestures with her hands. She was able to ask the doctors and nurses appropriate questions or suggest questions that Mara should ask.

Another one of Mara's friends, Mikala, visited with her mother. Mikala's mother, a slender, dark-complexioned lady who was visiting from

Grenada, said to Denise, "I am so sorry to see you in the hospital. Your face looks good though. You do not look sick."

"Thank you." Denise said smiling. "You and Mikala look like sisters."

Mikala laughed. Another, Pria with a broad smile on her face, walked into room. She wore scrubs as though she was coming from work.
"Hello Ms. Mitchell. This is my husband Robert," she said in her distinctive Kenyan accent.
Robert walked in behind her holding his hands down at his sides. He wore jeans and a plaid shirt. He had a very bright smile.

"Hello Ms. Mitchell. I'm sorry that you're not well," he said.

His accent was American. He and Pria stood shoulder to shoulder about same height. Pria then said, "Is it okay for us to say a prayer?" Denise said, "Yes, please."

Pria bowed her head and said, "Lord, we thank you for today. We trust that you will bless Ms. Mitchell and provide total healing. We know that you are a good God, and we look forward to her recovery. In Jesus name. Amen."   Ania visited as well, walking upstairs from her job, as she worked part-time at that hospital. She was wearing a black pair of pants, a beige blouse, and a white lab coat. She was light brown in complexion, slender, and she wore her curly black hair pinned up. She smiled. She said, "hello" in a soft voice to Denise. She gave both Denise and Mara a hug. She then walked over to the bedside and placed a gift bag on the table. The visitors took turns to be in the room, as this was the intensive care unit, and a limited number of visitors could be in the room at the same time. Denise was in good spirits. She did not feel isolated or abandoned. The back pain was persistent but the fact that her activities were limited helped to minimize movement and did not allow for any aggravation of the pain.

Chapter 5

Plan to Discharge

On November 30, 2016, after spending a few days in the critical care unit, at approximately 8:30 in the morning, Denise called her daughter.

"Mara, I need you to pick me up later when you get off work. They are discharging me."

"What do you mean they are discharging you? Did they say what is wrong?"

"The doctor said that he thinks it is muscular. He told me to take Tylenol and tramadol. They should help."

"You mean the same Tylenol and Tramadol you were taking before you went in? What kind of craziness is this? Mummy can you ask the doctor to give me a call please?"

"He left. He is probably seeing other patients."

Seething quietly, Mara admired how thoughtful her mother was in this situation.

"Okay…Tell your nurse to ask the doctor to give me a call." Mara said, trying to maintain her composure.

"Okay. Everything is okay with you?" Denise asked, trying to break the tension she could sense growing in her daughter's voice. "How's your morning going?"

"Yes, everything is fine, Mummy. It looks like it will be a busy day. I will check on you later. Love you."

"Love you too." Denise said.

***

Mara knew her mother was never one to disagree with medical professionals whom she trusted and expected to have interest in the best outcome for her. They were the experts, she felt, so she would listen and not say much. Even when she had questions, she was the type of patient that some nurses would refer to as a 'good patient.' She smiled even when she had pain. She did not want to "bother" the staff. In fact, in any setting, she was not one to intentionally try to ruffle feathers. However, Mara was less inclined to be trusting—given her own experience in the health care system.

About an hour after that conversation with her mother, Mara received a call from the attending physician. She was appreciative of the call because it was a courtesy on his part. Her mother was competent, and he could have told her to simply relay the information to her daughter. Although that was the usual practice, Mara knew that sometimes patients were, for several reasons, intimidated and hesitated to ask questions, because they knew they might not have a clear understanding of the explanations provided to them. Sometimes, too, physicians were in and out of the room so quickly that there was no opportunity to ask questions. Unfortunately, the health care system's business model, is overwhelmed. Physicians see too many patients in one day. But of course, that was not his fault. Mara was pleased that he took time to call.

"Your mother is probably experiencing muscular pain," the physician told her candidly. "I'm discharging her with a prescription for outpatient therapy as well as Tylenol and Tramadol for pain."

Mara listened carefully and realized that he did not have a valid explanation for her mother's pain.

"I really don't agree with that plan," Mara said, concluding that it was necessary to assert her opinion. "I think it's unsafe," she continued.

"My mother has been taking Tylenol and Tramadol and they have not been effective, so I

don't think that discharging her with the same medications will help."

There was an audible silence on the other
end.

"I really think we need to figure out what
the problem is," Mara reiterated. "She had an aortic dissection six years ago."

Mara expected that he knew this but felt
that she had to say it. She did not want her mother
to be at home and have a medical emergency without anyone else there with her. At least Mara had
been with her on that other occasion, six years prior,
when she had an aortic dissection. Given her mother's medical history, she thought, the physician
needs to order diagnostic tests. She did not see that
it made sense to discharge her mother with the
same medications that she had been taking prior to
admission. Denise was not a person who complained about pain just because she wanted to complain. She did not have any interest in continuously
taking medications. Like any other person, she wanted answers to the cause of the back pain, and she
wanted relief from it. The physician eventually said,
"I'll take another look to see if I missed something."

Second consult

A few hours later, Mara received another call from the attending physician with more information.

"I requested a second vascular surgery consult. The vascular surgeon requested the CT scan that was done in June of this year at the Washington Hospital. There is a 4cm difference noted in the scan that was done at the Washington Hospital from the one that we had done here at the Northern Metropolitan Hospital. Your mother is still dissecting. The vascular surgeon thinks that whenever your mother complains of back pain, there is a possibility that her aorta is dissecting. The dissection she had six years ago was in the ascending aorta. This time she is experiencing an aortic dissection in the descending part of the aorta. We will have to keep her here and treat her with medical management."

"A diagnosis!" Mara thought to herself. Understandably, there was also a mixture of relief and frustration. Before long, a flood of thoughts entered her mind: Why would they discharge her without checking further? What if she had not been suspicious? What if she did not ask those questions? What if she had not known what questions to ask? What if the doctor had decided her mother was over eighteen and did not need anyone else speaking for her? What if she had not been working in health care herself and not felt a sense of intimidation in contact with medical personnel? What if ...? All of this was very alarming.

But no ... it would be better to focus on the relief. She was relieved that there was an explanation for her mother's pain. She would hold on to the prescription for outpatient therapy that the doctor had given to her mother, but she would focus now on the present reality. She could not ignore her unease about the fact that she could have simply dropped her mother off at home if she had accepted the facility's assessment without question. But now ... her mother was experiencing another aortic dissection!

***

Denise's back pain persisted. The staff was treating her for pain and high blood pressure. Mara continued to communicate with her day and night. Of course, she continued with the job by which she made a living. She continued to review her patients' records and to make discharge planning arrangements for them. Trying to make sure that she ordered home services for one of her patients, while her mother remained on her mind. She requested home nursing, physical therapy, occupational therapy, and a home health aide from the home care agency representative on site for her patient. She tried to stay focused, but it was difficult, not knowing her mother's status. She avoided calling the hospital for updates and merely relied on her mother to give her information.

Daily, while she was at work, she corresponded with her mother by text messages and phone calls.

Mara: How are you feeling?

Denise: My back was hurting. I got some pain medication.

Mara: Oh. I'm sorry. Did you go to bed?

Denise: Yes, does not take me long, but up since 4. Catch up later.

Every evening, after work, Mara visited her mother and got more updates from the nurses while she was at her mother's bedside. As she sat at her mother's side, a young Caucasian woman in light blue scrubs walked into the room. Her blonde hair was in a short ponytail. She walked closer to Denise, smiled, and changed the IV bag.

"Hi. I'm Mara. I'm her daughter."

"Hello. I'm Erica. How are you?"

"I am okay, thanks. How is she doing? "

"She is doing okay. Her blood pressure fluctuates. She told me that you are a nurse," Erica replied, glad to speak to a fellow nurse. "I gave her hydralazine once today for the blood pressure. It seemed to have helped a little.

"Okay. Thanks. Hopefully, we can get this blood pressure under control soon," Mara said. "Are the doctors saying anything?"

"So far, they are not making any changes to the plan of care. Okay, nice meeting you." Erica said politely before leaving the room.

Mara continued to sit next to her mother's bed. Denise dozed off to sleep. Mara kissed her mother's forehead, and then left for the evening.

***

On December 3, 2016, Mara received a call from her mother, but responded with a text message, "Can I call you back? I am in report. Are you ok?" Her mother responded, "Yes. Was worried about you. Sure. I am fine."

If that, was it, worrying about Mara, there really was not anything to worry about, but that was Denise's personality. She worried about everything and everyone.

Mara returned her mother's call. They spoke about her vital signs, which were fluctuating, the persistent back pain, and how frustrated her mother was about being on bedrest. After completing her workday, Mara visited her mother, who was in good spirits and eager to get updates about the outside world. She asked about her family, friends, news from her job and her daughter's day.

On December 4th, the next afternoon, knowing that her mother remained on bed rest with bathroom privileges, Mara sent her a text, "Doing ok?"

Denise responded, "Just weak. That darn medication."

"Don't forget to call when you have to go to the bathroom," Mara said. "I am guessing they want you to drink a lot of fluids."

"Therein lies the problem."

All Mara could say was, "Sorry." She knew how frustrating all of this had to be for her mom.

By the time Mara saw her mother later that day, friends from Denise's job crowded the hospital room. The patient was in a jovial mood. She inquired about colleagues from the local offices, as well as about others in Chennai, India.

After about a week of medical management, the surgeon suggested to Denise and Mara, that surgery was the only other option to treat the aortic dissection. The broad-shouldered, six feet three inches tall surgeon, pulled a chair next to Denise's bed. He sat down and began describing a two-part procedure. The plan was to have the first part of the procedure done to repair the aorta at the thoracic area and a few days later, he would place a stent.

In preparation for surgery, the staff transferred Denise to a different unit on the same floor of the hospital. By then she knew all of the nursing assistants, nurses, housekeeping personnel and dietary personnel who had attended to her on the first unit. Mara was at her mother's bedside when Denise spoke to the nursing assistant.

"Hannah, will you come to visit me?"

"Of course, Ms. Mitchell," Hannah responded.

They both smiled. This was by no means unusual for her. She was a people-person. On the afternoon of her unit change, her friends from the first unit visited her and reassured her that she would have a good outcome from surgery. She was a woman of faith, as she always made clear, but she also had very human fears. She had an aortic dissection before, after which she was on the ventilator and sedated for over a week. Now, she feared a similar outcome.

Again, Denise's visitors continued to show support. Her friends Myra and Petra from two different workplaces, current and previous jobs, were at their friend's bedside. Myra brought nail polish as Denise requested that someone does her pedicure while she recovered. She joked about not wanting to have dry skin during her recovery. Her friend Nora traveled from New Jersey, so that she would be present to support Denise and Mara. In addition, she said, she thought that her own worry would be less if she were closer.

Now, the only thing left to do was wait.

Chapter 6

Surgery

December 7, 2016, was the day of surgery. Mara and Nora arrived at Denise's bedside just before 6am. Denise was wide awake as she had received a phone call an hour earlier from her friend Mable, who lived in Florida. Mable told Denise that she would like to pray with her prior to her procedure and Denise agreed. They were finished praying before her daughter and her friend arrived. As Mara and Nora sat at the bedside and talked with Denise, a very pleasant lady from the environmental services department, who had met Denise on the other unit, entered the room saying, "morning, morning."

In her green uniform, moving with slim grace, she walked over to her new friend, gave her a hug, and said with a Jamaican accent, "you'll be alright." On her way to work, she quickly left. She had just quickly visited to give good wishes. Five minutes later, the anesthesiologist, transporter and one of the operating room nurses arrived. The anesthesiologist spoke. He said, "Good morning, young lady. I am Dr. Bentley with anesthesiology.

This is Karen, the nurse and Dave with transport. Please tell me your name and date of birth." Denise looked up at him. She smiled. She said, "Denise Mitchell, July 2nd, 1955." He looked at her ID band. He said, "Okay. What are we doing today?" She sighed. "An aortic repair" she said. He told her, "Okay. I'll give you a little sedative through your IV. You will start feeling sleepy, but you will have enough time to get your hugs and kisses from your folks before you fall asleep. Then we will take you into the operating room." The tall slender nurse wore light blue scrubs, a cap and shoe covers. She turned to Nora and Mara. She said, "You guys can come with us on the elevator and then you can wait in the waiting area on the second floor." Nora smiled. She held Denise's hand, she prayed "Lord please bring her back to us safely." She kissed her on the forehead, "Good luck, girlie." Denise smiled, "Thank you." Mara kissed her mother on the cheek, "Good luck mummy. See you soon." Denise drifted off to sleep.

As Mara and Nora waited, Mara received a call from her friend Anita who said that she was on her way to sit with her in the waiting room. Anita arrived. The three sat patiently waiting for an update from the surgeon. As they waited, they did not say much. Mara thought, each was praying silently, expecting the best news and being thankful to God for his mercies. At noon, they had lunch in the cafeteria and then headed back to the waiting room. After approximately 6 hours of waiting, the tall vascular surgeon, Dr. Sam, came around the corner. His long legs just glided him over to where they sat. What he told them was the best news for Mara to be able to convey via group text messages to her mother's family and numerous friends. Surgery went well; there were no surprises. The surgical team transferred her mother back to her room on the critical care unit. Denise remained on the ventilator for the rest of the evening.

Chapter 7

Post-operative care

On December 8, 2016, the following morning, the medical team weaned Denise off the ventilator, and she breathed on her own. Later that evening, in a faint voice, she rated her pain level from a scale of zero to ten. She said that her pain was a four out of ten. She took her medications from her nurse by mouth, with apple sauce. It was a happy moment. Group text messages continued. Everyone who was connected to Denise in some way, was interested in her progress.

On December 9, 2016, mid-morning of the next day. Mara and Nora walked into what they quickly concluded was the wrong room at the Northern Metropolitan Hospital. There was a nurse in the room. As Mara thought about leaving quietly, the nurse said "Mara, I am so sorry." It was odd, Mara thought, that she was saying sorry when she was where she needed to be, but they were not where they were supposed to be. The nurse continued, "we had to put her back on the vent."

Mara did a double-take. They were in fact in the correct room. Her mother was on the ventilator, unrecognizable. Denise was swollen, with her tongue protruding out of her mouth. Shocked, Mara stood open-mouthed, looking at the shape on the bed that she now knew was her mother. She had received no phone call to prepare her for this. What happened? What could have caused her mother to look like this?

"What medication are you giving her?" Mara asked the nurse. "Did you give her medication?" The nurse answered, "Losartan."

This medication, Mara knew, doctors used to treat hypertension. She also knew that her mother had not taken that medication before. Her own nurse's training told her that the drug could be the culprit. It could cause this reaction—angioedema, significant swelling in Denise's face, tongue, and lips. It was a rare reaction from losartan; however, Mara knew enough to realize that it was possible. Simultaneously, her mother was also reacting to heparin, which resulted in heparin induced thrombocytopenia. This is a potentially life-threatening condition resulting from heparin therapy complications. In this case, heparin does the opposite of what it is supposed to do. It results in low platelet count and forms blood clots rather than preventing new blood clots, its intended purpose.

All of this went through Mara's thoughts as she watched her mother, who was so swollen that her eyes were closed shut. As Mara watched her mother, professional training, and familial fright and worry converged. In her head, she was nurse and daughter.

Calling this a setback would be an under-statement. This was a vastly different person lying in the bed. She had gone from taking her medications by mouth with applesauce the previous evening, to a state where now even her daughter had not initially recognized her. Scared and upset to see her mother in that condition, Mara asked follow-up questions.

"When did this happen? And why was she on heparin?" She asked. "She should not be on he-parin. She had already told the doctor about the reaction that she had with heparin."

"After she reacted to the medication around nine o'clock this morning, we put her back on the vent. I do not know anything about her not needing to be on heparin. The doctor ordered it," the nurse replied, glancing over her shoulder while hanging an IV bag.

Mara looked down at her mother, then back to the nurse, "I did not get a call about this. Does Dr. Sam know about her reaction to the medications?"

At this point, the nurse practitioner entered the room. "You did not get a call because it just happened—and yes Dr. Sam knows. We put her on the ventilator to protect her airways."

Mara turned slightly to look at the nurse practitioner whom she had seen on the unit the previous day. She took in the woman's crisp white uniform, the calm expression on her face, the brown eyes scanning the room. Mara was annoyed by how perfect she looked. She turned her attention back to her mother, her mouth slightly open, still in shock. She shook her head in disbelief and upset.

As she watched her mom, it did not take long to realize that two different timelines were given from the nurse and the nurse practitioner about when her mother was placed on the ventilator. One had said nine o'clock. The other said it had just happened. Something was not right. Was there a sense that they had to do damage control? Mara saw no point in prolonging the discussion. She was very worried about her mother.

***

The new focus at the hospital now was to keep Denise on the ventilator to protect her airway and to provide treatment for blood clots that were in Denise's neck, chest, and arms. The doctors placed her on another blood thinner, argatroban, to treat the blood clots. In the subsequent days, Denise had a series of procedures to remove the blood clots. Worried, Mara did not know what to do other than continue sending multiple group text messages to provide updates to friends and family and to request prayers.

Care for angioedema and heparin induced thrombocytopenia

Mara continued to visit her mother every day. While she was at work, she called daily to speak with the nurse or physician who was assigned to her mother. She wanted updates. She wanted to know what they were doing.

It was exactly two weeks after the initial reaction from losartan. From work, Mara called the nurse Katie, who was assigned to care for her mother, to get an update on Denise's condition. In their conversation, Katie the nurse, told Mara that the previous nurse had given her mother losartan. Mara paused. She was not certain that she had heard Katie correctly.

"I am sorry. What did you say?" Mara asked, feeling her heartbeat rapidly.

"Sorry," Katie, responded. "Your mom received losartan last night. It was ordered and the nurse did not realize that it caused the first reaction and so she gave it."

Mara was in disbelief. She thought, this is not possible. She wondered if there was any communication among the multidisciplinary team about patient care, particularly her mother's care.
"You got to be kidding me," She said to Katie. "I cannot believe this. I do not think this is even possible."

"I am so sorry," Katie said again. "Your mother is stable and apart from receiving losartan, there were no changes in her condition."

Mara was at work, with responsibilities there. She would have to wait until she got off from work to see her mother, especially since the official information was that Denise was stable. She would not be excused from her responsibilities at her own job to visit her mother. Containing her anger and disbelief, conscious that she would have to depend on hospital personnel for honesty and important updates, Mara thanked Katie for the update. She told her that she would be there to see her mother later in the evening after work. She had to be careful. They were the ones in charge of care.

She remained at work for seven more hours after the conversation with Katie. She worried about her mother for the entire day.

***

Mara arrived at her mother's bedside at six o'clock that evening. Her mother's face and arms were slightly more swollen than they had been the previous evening—which was very upsetting.

Ten minutes after Mara's arrival, the surgeon, Dr. Sam, entered Denise's room. He smiled and said to Mara, "hello." Worried and upset, Mara found it difficult to smile.

"Hello…I understand that my mother received losartan *again*. I cannot tell you how surprised, upset, disappointed, and worried I am." Mara said, not mincing words.

"I know—she won't receive it again," Dr. Sam said as he leaned against Denise's bedrail. "In fact, the order was discontinued, so the nurses won't give it to her again."

Mara's blank stare communicated that she wasn't impressed nor satisfied with his explanation. She was rapidly processing all the information she knew, about her mother's condition and what the providers discussed before. So, the order had *not* been discontinued prior to this…and that was written clearly in her mother's files. "What does one say in circumstances such as these?" She wondered. Even knowing and working within the health system, she realized, she did not know how to protect her mother.

"Do you have any questions?"

"No."

"Have a good evening," he said, quickly leaving the room.

So that was it? Honesty, but no real acknowledgement of error? Was *that* the most one could hope for? Did it make sense to show your dissatisfaction when you remained dependent on the facility's care?

While at work, Mara continued to call daily for updates regarding her mother's status. There was no change, but she remained hopeful. She visited her mother every evening after work. Although the staff sedated Denise while she was on the ventilator, and unable to provide any type of response, Mara spoke to her mother continuously. The staff at the hospital, seeing her visit all the time, expressed their worry for Mara and suggested that she take a break from visiting. She appreciated their concerns but saw no need to be anywhere else other than at her mother's side, every evening after work, to support her. The staff, she felt, would not understand. She had a strong bond with her mother. But quite apart from that, they themselves did not inspire confidence. How could she trust them to do what was best?

Mara and her mother spent a great deal of time doing various things together when her mother was well. Together, they attended church, shopped, visited family and friends, and traveled when they could. As her mother lay ill on a hospital bed, Mara could not think that there was anything else that required her attention or any other place that she needed to be. This was not the time to abandon her mother. When she was off from work, she visited earlier in the day and spent more time at her mother's side. Even if Denise were ill and appeared unresponsive, Mara believed her mother could hear her every word and she felt compelled to continue to visit and provide her with updates from the outside world. She wanted to be her cheerleader, to provide companionship and to ensure that her mother did not feel as though she was alone.

Three days after Mara had spoken with Dr. Sam, the multidisciplinary team was rounding at a time when Mara was visiting her mother. It was her day off from work. The team consisted of the surgeon's partner, nurse practitioner, educator, charge nurse, and nurse. Mara thought it was so nice that the charge nurse, Amy, walked into

Denise's room and asked her to participate in "rounds." This was a discussion held outside of the room. Mara agreed to attend. The physician presented the medical plan, then the nurse presented, explaining that lisinopril, an ace inhibitor used to treat high blood pressure and heart failure, had been ordered by the doctor and administered to Denise by the nurse. Listening, Mara was alarmed. She knew that, unfortunately, this medication could cause the same allergic reaction that losartan could cause. The swelling that Mara had observed on her mother had noticeably worsened and now that she heard about the administering of lisinopril, she understood the cause of the increased swelling. She interrupted the nurse's report and said, "Excuse me? Did you say she received lisinopril?" She had a profoundly serious expression on her face as she stared at each member of the team who was present. The entire team was embarrassed as no one made eye contact with Mara, except the surgeon. She thought that they were wishing that she, whom they had invited to attend rounds, was not present. The nurse responded, "Yes, she did." The physician then asked Mara if she had any other questions. She responded, "I have a statement, not a question. Please list all ARBS and Ace-inhibitors as allergies for my mother. That swelling will never go away if she continues to get these medications." The covering surgeon told Denise's nurse to add those classes of medications to the list of allergies. The nurse continued to speak and described the incision of the surgical site on Denise's chest and indicated that it was clean and dry, there was no bleeding or signs of infection such as redness and swelling noted by the nurse. The nurse also spoke about the tube feeding that the dietician had recommended. Denise tolerated the feeding well through her nostril without any nausea, vomiting or diarrhea. There were no further comments by other members of the team or by Mara. Charge nurse Amy told the group that there was nothing else to discuss about Denise and they would meet again to discuss her care on the following day. Amy, with a smile on her face, thanked Mara for attending. Mara nodded, thanked them as well and returned to her mother's bedside.

Mara was appalled. Did this always happen at hospitals? Was she particularly aware of it now because this was her mother? She thought about the places she had worked and the information to which she had access. She had never been this alarmed, as far as she could remember. Usually, hospitals had a pharmacy department and there would be at least one pharmacist that physicians had access to. Physicians, if they were not familiar with the medications that they ordered, would consult the pharmacist. It could even be helpful if a pharmacist would be present during the rounds as they discussed the patients' plan of care. While there would not have been any guarantee that lisinopril would have caused an allergic reaction, there was no reason to gamble with Denise's life, with the knowledge that the two medications could cause the same reaction. Denise's health condition was already compromised, and the physicians and nurses had an opportunity to rectify the situation that they had created for her, not make matters worse. She knew all of this from her experience in the nursing profession. She had learned a lot on the job. Why wouldn't they know these things too? Was she more attentive now because this was her mother? She thought, I hope I pay more attention to my patients and would not do things like this.

While Mara appreciated the fact that her mother was at what everyone agreed was a reputable hospital, she felt that she needed to be fully involved in her care. She reflected those errors could occur at any location. She thought now that those hired into direct patient-care positions may not necessarily have an interest in preserving the institution's reputation, or even the lives of individuals under their care. Her mother was on the critical care unit; however, the surgeon remained the attending physician. While the surgeon may have done an excellent job with the operation, Mara felt that the intensivist, who is the physician responsible for patients in the intensive care unit, should have taken over as the primary provider at that point, rather than someone who had repeatedly ordered medications that could potentially be fatal for her mother. In the interest of patient safety, the multidisciplinary team would have a meaningful involvement in every patient's care. She wondered now whether their involvement in Denise's case was standard procedure. She should not have had to make mention of the medication allergies during their rounds. What if she had not had information about these medications and about general procedure?! Would they continue to administer medications to her mother that were harmful to her? If the physician had not completed a medication reconciliation prior to the day that the staff observed the initial allergic reaction, the reaction should have prompted the completion of the medication reconciliation. A medication reconciliation is the process of ensuring that the patient's medication list is up to date. It would include the patient's allergies to help to prevent administration of harmful medications. Knowing about this from her own work within the system, it seemed to Mara that the providers may have omitted this process in Denise's case. Mara wondered if the nurses functioned as robots and did not have the ability to think about orders that they were conducting. As a nurse, she did not think the doctors infallible. It was standard procedure to listen, to question, to realize that the doctors were professionals who had studied to get where they were and could make mistakes. Did the doctors believe that the same medications worked the same way for all their patients? What role did nurses feel they could play? Did some hospitals have a good reputation simply because people did not know key details about care? Would she have imagined that the facility was doing what they should be doing if she had not had working experience of hospital care? These were worrying considerations.

The intensivist scheduled a family meeting. The attendees expected to be present were the intensivist, the surgeon, nurse, charge nurse, Aunt Breana, and Mara. There was some miscommunication and so the surgeon was unable to attend. It would have been helpful to have the surgeon present at the meeting, to have clarity on his approach to delivery of care.

The meeting was held with the intensivist Dr. Miles, the charge nurse Amy, Aunt Breana, Mara and Janie, Denise's goddaughter, a medical school graduate, who was visiting her from Boston. Mara reflected that it was a good thing there were health professionals among her mother's family and friends. Aunt Breana and Mara requested to have Denise's care transferred to the intensivist team. Families, Mara thought, should not have to make those suggestions. If all were going well, that would not be an issue; however, in this case, there were medical issues for the doctors to address and should not overlook. Both Mara and Breana were in the health field, and both were alarmed.

In this meeting, the family discovered from Dr. Miles that Denise had suffered a few strokes. They only found out because Breana and Mara asked that question. Denise's left hand, they noted, was very swollen. In response to commands by nurses and doctors, Denise was unable to move the hand. However, three days before the family meeting, when both Mara and Aunt Breana asked the surgeon if Denise had a stroke, the surgeon said, "no."

He said that the hand was too heavy for Denise to lift due to fluid overload. Now, Dr. Miles the intensivist, discussed the result of a CT scan which showed that Denise had suffered a stroke that affected her left side. So, Mara wondered, was the surgeon trying to conceal the truth about the strokes? It was unclear why he would want to do this. Now she could no longer avoid comparisons or find excuses. There was a vast difference between this experience and the 2010 experience, when Denise had had a stroke. Mara reflected that the physician could have been truthful about the fact that Denise had suffered a stroke and if he were uncertain, he should have sought a second opinion. The outcome of not sharing information that

Denise had a stroke was denial of services, primarily therapy, which was vital for her recovery.

As Dr. Miles informed them about radiology reports, they learned that the CT scan showed a subarachnoid hemorrhage. This condition is characterized by a bulging blood vessel that bursts in the brain. It is a serious condition that may lead to brain damage or death. Another CT scan result reported possible watershed infarcts, which is a condition in which there is a blockage of blood flow to an area of the brain. It is located at the farthest point of blood supply from two separate cerebral arterial systems. Dr. Miles also discussed an EEG that the team conducted on Denise. This is a test used to evaluate the electrical activity of the brain. The EEG indicated that Denise had seizure activity, although no one had witnessed a seizure. Dr. Miles informed the family that the nurses and doctors would maintain Denise on seizure precautions. These precautions included closely monitoring her and placing soft padding against her bedrails to protect her from hurting herself if she had a seizure.

The family meeting ended. Dr. Miles offered to be available by phone if they had any further questions later. Of all the things they talked about, Mara reflected, she had known about one—the EEG. On the afternoon on which it was conducted, she had arrived on her mother's unit and met four of her mother's coworkers who had mentioned that they would visit and pray at her bedside. They were truly kind, and genuinely concerned about their friend. Enid had been in contact with Mara prior to this meeting. She introduced the other ladies in the group. Denise had spoken well of all of them, Mara recalled. And she was very fond of the youngest, Anna, who said how much she missed seeing her friend in the office. Mara saw that her mother's colleagues really cared about Denise.

As she continued to reflect on her mother's care, Mara could not help but wonder about the care that her mother was receiving at the hospital. What was happening? Did the hospital really have a plan for the care of her mother, or any real interest in her recovery? Now she asked herself the question that was important to her as both a professional and a daughter—did these facilities really *care* about patient care?

Chapter 8

Tracheostomy and gastrostomy

It was several weeks since Denise had allergic reactions from the two medications losartan and heparin, but the swelling in her face, neck, lips, and tongue were still present. She was still on the ventilator. The physicians spoke to Mara about placing a tracheostomy, which is an opening in the trachea through the neck to allow the movement of air.

"Your mom has been on the vent for several weeks now," Dr. Miles called Mara to explain. We need to put a tracheostomy and place a feeding tube. Just letting you know as we need to get consent."

"Okay, sure," Mara said thinking, the tracheostomy and feeding tube would be okay as it is just temporarily.

The tracheostomy would, she imagined, also give Denise's swollen tongue and lips a chance to heal. The ventilator would then be connected to the tracheostomy. Mara also thought about the feeding tube, called a gastrostomy tube, which would be placed in her mother's stomach. That would replace the tube in Denise's nostril through which she was being fed.

"Okay. If you are agreeing, let me get the nurse on the line to witness."

Nurse, Jessica, came on the line, "Hello, this is Jessica. To whom am I speaking?" Mara responded, "This is Mara Mitchell."

"Hi Mara," Jessica continued, "Are you agreeing to have the tracheostomy and peg tube placed for your mom, Denise Mitchell?"

"Yes," Mara replied.

"Okay. Thank you." Jessica acknowledged, before they ended the call. The physician placed the tracheostomy and feeding tube on January 11th, 2017.

Chapter 9

Blood pressure management

During the same period when the intensivist informed Mara of the report of possible watershed infarcts, Denise's blood pressure was consistently elevated. The blood pressure issue was a big concern because Denise had vascular surgery and it was imperative to maintain normal blood pressure so that it did not affect the surgical site or worse, provoke another dissection. In addition, given the fact that she had experienced a few strokes, the neurologist was also involved and did not want her blood pressure to be too low. It became a matter of maintaining a medium somehow between the vascular surgeon and the neurologist. Denise was placed on three different drips to normalize the blood pressure; yet the systolic blood pressure had readings over two hundred. Normal blood pressure is a reading below 120/80. Hers was 200s/100s. Mara and Aunt Breana suggested to the staff that, to obtain a more accurate reading, they should measure the blood pressure with a manual cuff and not with the monitor. The staff did not do as requested. Mara did not know what the rationale was for ignoring the request.

The staff kept Denise on the propofol drip which is normally used for sedation. In her case, the nurses used this medication also to manage her blood pressure. At least, this was the explanation given to Mara by one of her mother's nurses, Emily. The nurses also medicated Denise for pain with dilaudid. That, Mara thought, was a significant amount of medication for someone who, before that hospitalization, she had not been taking many medications, apart from her blood pressure and acid reflux medications.

Mara, a daughter first—but also a registered nurse, wanted to see her mother's health improve. While she did not want to step on anyone's toes, she could not ignore the issues presented. Mara's observation of all this made her continue to question all that she thought she knew about nursing. As she watched the way the nurses cared for her mother, she reflected that in her experience critical thinking on the part of nurses was an important part of the process. Nurses were taught to advocate for patients, and she hoped to observe this skill in her mother's care. If there was any doubt, she hoped that the nurses would question orders prior to carrying them out.

She could not imagine that nurses would administer medications, and *then* question the orders. What she was witnessing seemed to be a 'shoot first and ask questions later' type of approach. There was, she felt, no logic to that type of thinking. She wondered if the nurses felt intimidated by the physicians and afraid to do what they thought was right— or was it that they did not know what was right, and did not think they had the authority to question or try to find out? She also wondered if the nurses and physicians felt as though they had already done the damage and they had no interest in struggling with the patient. Were they asking themselves why bother?

Mara could not get away from the thought that her mother's condition was because of a reaction to a medication, that it had been worsened by a later administration of the same and then a similar medication. It was not a situation in which the doctors had diagnosed Denise with a terminal illness and her daughter was in denial. She is ill, yes, Mara reflected, but she should be taken care of properly. She had survived the aortic dissection. She survived! It was post-surgical care that resulted in catastrophes. Mara wanted to see ownership of the fact that Denise had received improper care. They needed to take accountability. She wanted those who were responsible and others who participated in her mother's care to treat her mother with dignity and acknowledge that she wanted to live and that her family wanted her to live as well. She wanted it acknowledged that, although she had a serious condition, her mother had been doing well until the hospital made mistakes. Mara would have liked to just be a daughter to her mother and be able to visit without wondering about future mishaps, about the adequacy of the treatment given by the healthcare professionals, or about her own role in identifying a remedy.

Arterial line

On the morning of January 24, 2017, Mara had seen her mother's blood pressure at a high of 206/110. She was at work when a phone call came from the Northern Metropolitan Hospital. Mara promptly answered. It was the attending intensivist for the week, Dr. Cho.

"I would like to have an arterial line placed in your mother's arm to obtain a more accurate blood pressure measurement," He explained. "To do this, we need to have consent."

Mara listened and said, "Of course." She did not know what the hospital's protocol was, but she was aware that sometimes patients in the intensive care unit would have an arterial line in place and the staff would obtain blood pressure readings this way. Her mother may have had one placed pre-operatively and the providers removed it. After the radiologist placed the arterial line, Dr. Cho called Mara again and informed her, "Well the line is in. We have a more accurate blood pressure reading!"

It was nice that he had called back but she knew that she had planned to call anyway. With knowledge that she was a nurse he told her with excitement, "The systolic blood pressure from the arterial line is 100 points less than the reading from the monitor!"

It was understandable that he would be pleased. This discovery would eliminate the need to discover the cause of the elevated blood pressure and it also meant there was no need to increase the dosage of the current medications or to add other agents.

***

"I am not misinterpreting this. But I have to say it to myself so that I am clear. The new reading means that they were treating my mother for high blood pressure unnecessarily," Mara thought to herself.

In fact, she was being told now, her mother's blood pressure was low. And hadn't she and

Aunt Breana asked them to use another method that might be more effective? Mara could not help it and told Dr. Cho the assessment she made.

"So, all this time with her being on all these different meds, she was being treated unnecessarily for high blood pressure..."

Dr. Cho, of course, was busy. "I'm sorry," he told her. "I do have to see another patient.

I just wanted to give a brief call to fill you in."

And indeed, he had not been obliged to call. But there was no attempt at an explanation, no apology. The call was brief.

Was this real? Had they discovered a mistake and corrected it? Mara reflected that there was never a time for updates from the physicians except if she and her aunt Breana requested a meeting with Dr. Miles, the other intensivist. There was no doubt in Mara's mind now that other reports of worsened health, specifically multiple watershed infarcts on the CT scan as well as kidney impairment, resulted from the poor blood pressure management.

Alarmed and annoyed by all this, Mara understood that she did not require permission from anyone to advocate for her mother. She knew what was right. Her mother's care was not *care* at all. The hospital owed it to Denise to provide proper care or transfer her elsewhere—where safe and appropriate treatment would be provided to restore her mother's health. Afraid for her mother, Mara wondered what her options were. She wondered about the possibility of moving her mother to a tertiary care facility such as the University Hospital. Tertiary care facilities are more prepared with the expertise to manage complex cases. She thought that a transfer to an upper level of care would be justified and should be covered by her mother's health insurance company. Would it be?

***

Edema

As the days progressed, there was no improvement in Denise's condition. In fact, she seemed to have gotten worse. The swelling in the face and upper torso appeared to have worsened. Every few hours, the nursing staff turned her to her sides. The eye on the side to which they turned her, was swollen shut. Each time she visited; Mara had the feeling that the nurses had lost confidence in their own abilities to nurse their patient back to life —to something meaningful. Now, they were making comments to her suggesting this.

During one visit, Emily, the nurse in attendance, looked from Mara to her mother, with concern.

"I don't think she would want to live like that," she said.

Mara could feel the blood pounding in her temples. Like what? Did she honestly believe that Denise and her family had given up on life? Mara talked to her mother at her bedside every day, while she continued to be on the ventilator with her eyes closed.

"Mummy, you are still in the hospital. Blink your eye twice if you want to live."

Mara could still feel her heart beating fast even though it was only one minute that passed before seeing her mother respond. She watched carefully. Denise blinked her right eye twice. Denise was unable to do the same with the left eye; it was too swollen. At every request, Denise obliged and as requested, blinked the eye that remained opened.

***

From work, Mara called the Northern Metropolitan Hospital for an update. She spoke with Nurse Jessica.

"Your mom is more swollen than she was yesterday."

Mara gasped and then stared at the computer screen. She put her right hand to her forehead and held both of her temples. Mara closed her eyes for a moment. She spoke again to Jessica.

"What is happening? What do you mean? How can she be more swollen?" Mara said, as she got up from her desk and started down the hallway toward the waiting area.

"Apart from the swelling, she is otherwise stable. So, we will see you this evening?" Jessica said, seeming to be in a hurry.

"Yes. Okay thanks. Bye." Mara replied abruptly. They ended the call.

Everything that **Mara** knew or thought she knew about nursing seemed to be wiped clean from her brain. She put her phone in her pocket and sat on one of the chairs in the visitors' waiting area on the unit. With her elbows resting on her knees, she leaned forward and held her head in her hands. She quietly started praying, "Please Lord, take care of Mummy."

Mara's eyes filled with tears and she could no longer keep her composure. It was not long before Mara began to sob uncontrollably. In her mind she asked several questions. How could her mother continue swelling like that? What if she bursts open? Her face cannot just keep growing like that. What happens next? Will her eyes disappear?

Why are the physicians just allowing her condition to worsen and they are not making efforts to provide care that would improve her health? Because they can.

"I know they can do something," Mara whispered to herself.

Mara googled her mother's cardiologist and found his number, then called. His wife, who was also his secretary, picked up immediately and said in a friendly voice, "Dr. McKenzie's office."

"Good morning," Mara said, wiping away tears while also trying to keep her voice from quivering. "My name is Mara. My mom is Denise Mitchell and she is at Northern Metropolitan Hospital. Can I speak with Dr. McKenzie, please?"

"Oh! Yes dear." Mrs. McKenzie, replied probably still sensing some distress in Mara's voice. "I'll transfer you to him."

On the first ring, Dr. McKenzie responded with a loud voice, "Hello! How can I help you?" Mara was startled by the sound of his voice. Although she had met Dr. McKenzie before at one of her mother's appointments, it was her first conversation with him.

"Hi, Dr. McKenzie. My name is Mara. My mom, Denise Mitchell is at Northern Metropolitan Hospital," she said. Mara paused for a moment to prevent the floodgates of emotions from opening again. She continued, "My mother had another aortic dissection and had surgery to repair it. Then she had a few complications such as angioedema from losartan and heparin induced thrombocytopenia. She is back on the vent and several things have been happening to her. She is very swollen, and the swelling just keeps getting worse and worse. She is unrecognizable. I want her to transfer out of that hospital to the Washington Hospital or the University Hospital. Her issues are too complicated for them at Northern Metropolitan Hospital. I am looking for assistance to transfer her out."

"Well, I don't have privileges at that hospital," Dr. McKenzie said as he cleared his throat. To Mara his response sounded impatient and unconcerned. "It's true, my partner does have privileges," he continued.

"She can look in on your mom. Your mom is in a good place! Do not focus too much on the swelling—it is merely cosmetic. Do not worry about it." Dr. McKenzie said abruptly. "Alright hang in there! Bye now!" The call ended.

Mara sat looking down at her phone in disbelief. He had not sounded at all concerned. Mara continued her quest for help. She had her mother's primary care physician's card in her wallet and called his number. He did not pick up, so she left a voicemail message, "Hi Dr. Daniel. It's Mara, Denise Mitchell's daughter. She is at Northern Metropolitan Hospital, and I am looking for assistance to transfer her out of there. Can you please give me a call?"

Twenty minutes later, Mara received a call from Dr. Daniel. He was very friendly and noticeably sounded concerned. In a very calm voice, he said, "Hi Mara. It's Dr. Daniel. I'm sorry that your mom is in the hospital. You know, I do not have privileges there, so I will not be able to transfer her. You can talk to the people there at Northern Metropolitan Hospital to see if they will transfer her. I would not recommend her being transferred to where I am because it would be at the same level of care as where she is."

Feeling disappointed again, Mara said, "I did not want to talk to them about transferring her because I do not think they're even listening to anything that I say. I was hoping that another doctor could speak to them."

"Give it a little more time," Dr. Daniel replied. "Let us see how things go. Okay? Take care." His voice was soothing and more comforting in comparison to the other call. Realizing that there was not much else to say, Mara said, "Okay, thank you. Bye."

Not willing to give up in her efforts to have her mother transferred to a tertiary care hospital, Mara thought again of Dr. Jimmy, from all those years ago—2010, when her mother had the first aortic dissection. She googled the number of the facility where she thought she might find him. The secretary answered, speaking in a friendly voice, "Vascular surgery. How can I help you?"

"Hi, good morning…Can I speak with Dr. Jimmy please?"

"May I ask who's calling?"

Feeling confident at the chance to speak with Dr. Jimmy, Mara replied, "My name is Mara. I am calling on behalf of my mother Denise Mitchell, a former patient of his."

"He no longer works here," the secretary said. "But his partner does, so I can transfer you to her."

Mara was relieved that she could at least speak with his partner, "thank you."

"You're welcome. Hold for the transfer." The phone rang a few times, and a voicemail came on, "This is Dr. Jeffers. Please leave a message and I will get back to you at my earliest convenience."

Mara left a message, "Hi Dr. Jeffers. My name is Mara. I am calling on behalf of my mother Denise Mitchell, a former patient of Dr. Jimmy in 2010. She had an aortic dissection back in 2010 and had another one in November 2016. She is at Northern Metropolitan Hospital, and I am looking for assistance to transfer her to a tertiary care hospital. My number is 301-555-5555."

Within ten minutes, Mara received a call from Dr. Jeffers. She sounded concerned. "This is Dr. Jeffers. I am sorry I just missed your call. You said that your mom is a former patient of Dr. Jimmy? Tell me what is going on."

Mara explained, "Yes. Dr. Jimmy treated her in January 2010. She recently had an aortic dissection in the descending aorta and had surgery to repair it. Unfortunately, she had quite a few complications that started with angioedema from losartan and from heparin induced thrombocytopenia. She is having a lot of swelling that are getting worse and worse. I do not think that they are able to take care of her at Northern Metropolitan Hospital and I want her to be transferred."

Dr. Jeffers sounded empathetic, "I am so sorry to hear that. We will investigate to see if we can help. Dr. Jimmy does not work at the University Hospital anymore. I work with him at Greatland Hospital. If there is anything that we can do, we will contact you and the Northern Metropolitan Hospital. Okay? Take care."

For the first time in a long while, Mara was hopeful. As the call ended, she remained seated in the waiting area on her unit at the hospital where she worked and recalled conversations with her mother. Mara recalled her mother saying, "Dr. Jimmy is an excellent surgeon. He knows what he is doing."

The thought alone made Mara smile. That was much needed reassurance that the steps she had taken might make a real difference. Still, it did not take long for her mind to circle back to the current situation. Tears began to fall again. She could not contain her emotions. Her two friends Shantel and Becka were passing by separately and saw her sitting in the waiting area. They both approached and consoled her.

Becka, as she rested her hand on Mara's shoulder prayed, "Lord please watch over Mara's mom. Protect her. Give her the strength to keep fighting. Bless Mara and her entire family. I pray that they will have faith for her mother's healing. Thank you, Lord, for all your blessings. Amen."

Shantel sat next to Mara and placed her hand on Mara's arm. She said to Mara, "It is going to be okay. I know this is hard. Your mom is a tough lady." The three remained in the waiting area for ten more minutes and then Mara said, "Thank you. I better go wash my face and get back to work." The three walked back to the nursing unit.

Later that evening, Mara visited her mother. The eye that her mother had previously been able to open, now barely opened. The intensivist, Dr. Miles, who had listened to Mara and Breana, saw her at her mother's side and entered the room. She stood about five feet away from Mara, who was sitting next to her mother's bed. Dr. Miles had smiling eyes and kept her hands to her sides as she spoke to Mara. Her voice was soft and calm. She glanced over at Denise and then to Mara and said, "You are doing such a wonderful job supporting your mother. You know, this is how she is going to be. Do you think that she will want to live like this?"

Mara looked at her, bent to pick up a piece of tissue that had fallen to the floor. This must be the topic on the unit! Were they all just waiting for her to say that it would be okay to stop treating her mother? Well, she could not! She would not! They had made mistakes! It was infinitely possible for her mother to recover. Had not this same woman talked to them as if she were listening, as if…. The intensivist—what was her name? Suddenly Mara could not remember—she was speaking again.

"You know, some families would just take her off the ventilator and in a few days, she'll just pass away, peacefully."

A terminal wean? Is that what she is suggesting? That is the description of a terminal wean! Absolutely not! Pass away peacefully?

Dr. Miles! That was her name. What did she mean "peacefully?" A thousand thoughts flooded Mara's mind at once. Perhaps some pass away peacefully like that. Not my mother! I know her. You do not! She would die worrying. Worry is what she always does. And do you want her to die worrying? That is not what I want for my mother? This may be normal to you, Dr. Miles, but not to me. She is just another patient to you, as well as, to the other providers at the hospital. Absolutely not. This is my mother. My best friend. Someone's daughter. Someone's sister. Someone's grandmother. Someone's aunt. Someone's cousin. Someone's best friend. Someone's friend. Someone's colleague. Someone's employee.

"Dr. Miles, if it's a miracle I have to pray for, then that's what I will do." Mara responded.

Mara was constantly glancing over at her mother, remembering how she had talked about hearing what the nurses said in 2010 while she was on the ventilator with her eyes closed.

"She blinks her eye when I ask her to." Mara said, using this important nuance to support her reason for hope.

Dismissively shaking her head from side to side with a smirk of condescension, "It is what you are expecting but she is not actually responding," Dr. Miles said. "Okay. I will let you continue to visit. I will see you again."

"Did they actually say things like this to family members?" Mara wondered as she watched Dr. Miles walk away.

She remained seated on the chair next to her mother's bed. Mara turned to her mother, "Mummy, I am so proud of you. You are doing great. I believe that if you want to, you would be on your feet again. I do need you. I say that but I do not want to be selfish and would not force you to continue to fight if you are too tired and are ready to move on to the next world. Hopefully, you are not too tired of me asking you this, but I need to ask you again. If you want to live, please blink your eye twice." Although Denise, barely able to open her eye, Mara saw her mother blink her eye twice. She smiled and said, "Thanks Mummy."

Mara continued to send text messages to friends and family:

Hello everyone, mummy's vitals are stable, and labs are okay. She still has a long way to go with the swelling in her lips, tongue, and neck. Until that swelling goes down, she will remain on the vent. Thanks for all the prayers.

***

Denise's face was still swollen, or, as they would say in the profession, the edema was still present. The hospital used diuretics to remove excess fluid and the nurses also used pillows to elevate Denise's arms and legs to reduce and prevent any further swelling. Denise also needed the staff to turn her to her sides to help to prevent pressure ulcers.

One day, Mara walked into her mother's room and noticed that her swollen extremities were directly on the bed. Denise was lying flat on her back and the only pillow on the bed was the one underneath her head.

The nurse Amira walked into the room shortly after Mara arrived.

"What happened to her pillows?" Mara inquired.

"We're short of pillows on the unit."

We're short of pillows on the unit? Should she be bringing pillows from home? It was a pity the hospital had a shortage, but wasn't Denise a patient in particular need? Did they care so little that they could not take a pillow from another room? What was going on? Had they unilaterally decided it was all over? Mara wondered.

"I'm just concerned about her edema and pressure ulcers," Mara said directly.

A different nurse and nursing assistant who were standing outside of Denise's room, promptly went on a pillow search and returned with pillows to replace the ones that staff had taken away.

The nurse who was helping, placed the new pillows on top of the trash can while the nursing assistant proceeded to the other side of the bed to turn Denise. *On top of the trash can?* Mara was flabbergasted. Her eyes moved from the nurse back to the pillow. She could say something now, of course, but what kinds of things happened when she wasn't there? They had gone to search for pillows when they were not even assigned to Denise, so she felt sure they were not being malicious when they put the pillow on the trash can. *But what did this say about general practice?* Her eyes filled as she reminded herself that she was not at her mother's bedside twenty-four hours a day, seven days a week and was obviously unaware of all they were doing and not doing regarding her mother's care. Should she say something? How could she not? Mara paused, cleared her throat, tried to make sure her tone remained neutral.

"You know, I am really concerned about more complications and about her pillows being placed on the trash can and then placed on her bed. Why expose her to anymore?"

"The trash can is closed," The nurse argued. She was obviously not in a frame of mind to learn anything. Her tone suggested that she took the comment as an affront.

"Let's not use these pillows," Mara said quietly. "I am afraid of infections for her. Could you bring *clean* pillowcases please?"

The nurse did not respond but walked over to the cabinet, took out four pillowcases and handed them to Mara and slowly walked out of the room. Mara cleaned the pillows with the disinfecting wipes that were on the counter in the room and placed the pillows on her mother's bed. She looked over at the door and saw two nursing assistants standing there. She knew they were nursing assistants by the burgundy scrubs they wore. "Can you please help me?" Mara said. They both responded immediately, "Sure, we can help."

They were both slim young women, by their accents West African and Trinidadian. Both ladies were about same height five feet three inches tall. They were dark complexioned. They both wore braids in their hair. Perhaps they helped because Denise could have been their mother, or Mara could have been their sister. Either way, Mara needed the support, and they were there. The assistants turned Denise to the right side and Mara placed a pillow underneath her mother's lower back. She also elevated her mother's arms and legs with the other pillows. Denise was critically ill and unable to respond to express her discomforts.

If, Mara reflected, she did not have interest in her mother's wellbeing, whom could she expect to do so? Being a witness to such poor judgment by staff made Mara wonder about the type of care that staff provided in her absence. She thought that all she could do about that was to pray. She continued to send out group text messages to update family and friends and to request prayers for her mother's recovery. The hospital had an interesting way of making them all feel so helpless. It really was a good thing that many of Denise's friends and family had faith in the power of prayer.

Chapter 10

Hospice or dialysis

On January 27, 2017, as she went about her morning routine at work, Mara received a call from Dr. Kennedy, the intensivist who had just come on duty at Northern Metropolitan Hospital for the week.

"Your mother is not doing well," he explained to Mara. "I know you have been receiving updates. So, decisions regarding her care going forward, need to be made. Your mother is in multi-organ failure. She has an extremely poor prognosis and if she survives, she will not have a good quality of life."

Mara held the phone and sighed. With her eyes closed, she leaned her head back and opened her eyes to look at the ceiling. Feeling frustrated and uneasy with the information that the intensivist was giving her, she switched the phone to the other hand.

"You should consider hospice," Dr. Kennedy continued.

Was this, she wondered, a tactic used by the hospital? Did they think it was easier to have someone who had not yet established any sort of connection with the patient and her family be the one to be even more direct and uncaring? Or was this tone a tactic used by this individual?

Did he think he was talking about a pet to be taken to the veterinarian and put to sleep? To Mara, the intensivist's tone suggested that there was no reason to consider any alternatives but that, hospice. Mara sucked her teeth—quietly, so he wouldn't hear it, and this made her think that now she was in Caribbean mode. Whether or not he wanted to hear her opinion, she would let him have it.

She paused. "Do not cry, Mara," she thought to herself. "You know you do not communicate effectively when you cry. Hold it in."

She got up from her desk and started walking down the hallway of her hospital very quickly. She held the phone with her left hand and with her right hand, palm up, she gestured as she responded, "My 61-year-old mother walked into the emergency room with complaints of back pain. She has had a number of setbacks, no fault of hers, and you're quick to give up on her. What are the other options?"

"It's either dialysis or hospice."

Hospice! Was that all she could do? From what Mara knew, hospice was a good service if you were at the end of the road—if one's intention was to end treatment. She had not intended to end treatment for her mother.

"Then dialysis it is."

"All right then…thanks. Have a good day," the physician said, cutting the conversation short.

Why was it so possible for these people to tell you about the worst things in the calmest tone, then later say with equal calm and no conviction, "have a good day" Mara thought.

Later, as she sat at her desk at work, Mara reflected that if only she could have recorded those insensitive, waste of time conversations that she was forced to endure, she could listen to them repeatedly until they made some sort of sense. That was such a vast spectrum: dialysis or hospice. Had he not had a conversation or hand-off from his colleagues about Denise and her daughter? What would be his rationale to present those as options? It would have been reasonable if he had called Mara and informed her that her mother was in renal failure and needed to have dialysis. Mara would then have had an opportunity to accept or decline dialysis on her mother's behalf. Given the amount of interest that Mara had demonstrated in her mother's recovery, it was an easy decision that she would accept dialysis. She reflected on how they had been preparing her mother for an early discharge from Northern Metropolitan Hospital, without a diagnosis, yet with a prescription for outpatient therapy, Tylenol, and tramadol. Discharged! How can they now explain all that is happening? Does their documentation give a true account of what Denise had been through? Would they not be concerned and show significant interest not to continue to make poor decisions regarding her care? How can their approach to Denise's case indicate such lack of care and overt readiness to relinquish delivery of life sustaining methods, without regard for the patient's or family's goals of care? Was this about money? Or was it about something else? What was it?

Later that day, Mara visited her mother. Denise was lying on her back and so her right eye opened slightly. Mara put her bag down and pulled a chair up close to her mother's bed. She leaned over her.

"Mummy you are doing a fantastic job. Blink your eye twice if you want to live."

After about a minute, as Mara watched closely, she saw her mother's eyelid move twice. Mara smiled. She told her, "Your kidneys are not functioning properly, so you'll need to have dialysis."
There was no reaction, no change in expression from Denise. Mara continued to look

at her mother's face. She added, "They will insert a dialysis catheter perhaps tomorrow. I am not sure when and you will start dialysis soon."

Mara remembered from a previous conversation with her mother, that her mother was curious as to whether she was on dialysis from her first aortic dissection, six years prior. Denise had asked that question in 2010 because she remembered being told by the doctors at the University Hospital that her kidneys were not functioning well. At that time, Mara had told her mother no. They never discussed whether her mother would want to have dialysis if ever needed. Because now she senses a lack of response from her mother, Mara thinks, *after that first aortic dissection, I should have talked to her about what she would want and specifics about the advanced directive.*

Mara stopped talking. At this point, she was simply notifying her mother, who had already appointed her with the authority to make decisions on her behalf. She sat next to her mother in silence, thinking about life, thinking about how sudden all of this had been, wondering what her mother was thinking.

Chapter 11

Dialysis

On January 28, 2017, again, Mara was at her desk at work when she received a call from Northern Metropolitan Hospital. She immediately answered. It was one of the nurses, Heather, with an interventional radiologist, Dr. Thomas.

"We're calling to get consent for a dialysis catheter as your mom needs to start dialysis," the physician stated. "Just so you know, there are risks associated with the procedure. There is the risk of bleeding, infection, and air embolism. Are you giving consent?"

Mara stared at the wall in front of her. She was conscious that her expression must be blank as she said, "Yes, I'm giving consent."

"Okay, let me have you talk to Heather," the radiologist said.

"Hello Mara. Did you understand everything that Dr. Thomas said and are you giving consent?" The nurse said.

Mara rubbed her right temple and repeated, "Yes, I understand and I'm giving consent."

After about an hour and a half, Mara received another call from Heather, the nurse at Northern Metropolitan Hospital. Mara was walking down the hallway on the unit at her hospital. She picked up the phone and went to the far end of the hallway.

"Everything went well," Heather stated. "Your mom tolerated the procedure. She is heading back to the unit with the transport staff."

"Okay, thanks Heather."

Mara felt relieved. A feeling she had not felt in a long while.

***

The next morning, Denise started dialysis with no significant issues. Mara was off that day, so she drove directly to hospital to see her mother. As she stood at her mother's bedside, she noticed that her mother seemed weak. She was very sleepy and barely opened her eyes. Otherwise, there were no issues.

It was sixty four number of days since Denise entered the hospital. Mara began to take note of her mother's labs and vital signs. She would call her mother's nurse daily for updates and felt encouraged by the improvements that she started to notice, even if the care team failed to acknowledge these improvements. She questioned herself regarding the daily calls to the hospital. Should she wait until the end of the day when she arrived at the hospital to get updates? No! Too many hours to wait. How could she concentrate at work and not know about her mother's status? Feeling she must be a bother, she explained that to the nurses. They said they had no objections to providing her with lab results and vital signs. She was always grateful to some of the nurses for their kindness in taking time to give her updates. She was aware that they were busy, and that her mother was not their only patient, but without the information Mara would worry all day.

Mara consulted her aunt Ali, her mother's close friend in Maryland, who was a retired pathologist, as well as her mother's sister in Grenada, Simone, an emergency room physician. Both were very objective with the information that they provided to their niece. Of course, both were also interested in their niece's wellbeing. They wanted to make sure that she was eating properly and getting sufficient rest. Mara was eating. Her mother's friends Myra and Jenice brought an abundance of food for her, cooked food as well as grocery items. She had no excuse to not eat. Rest was a different matter. No one could bring that to her. If only they could, she thought, longing greedily for rest. She found it increasingly difficult to sleep, night after night.

Denise needed prayers to get through that storm. Being of Catholic faith, she usually would not miss mass if a ride were available to her. Since Mara worked every other weekend, they usually attended church together every other weekend. Now, Aunt Ali contacted the church and requested that a priest visit Denise. In addition, Denise's friend Lori, who was a member of the same church that she enjoyed attending, had her name placed on the prayer list. Every Sunday, the lector announced her name among the list of sick congregants. Some of her friends, including her friend Marge in Marietta, Georgia, dedicated services at their churches for her. At the hospital, the priest or someone from pastoral services visited her. She received the anointing of the sick. Denise's family and friends believed that prayers as well as determination to live allowed her to remain in the fight to survive.

Denise's friends who lived out of town in various states expressed feelings of frustration and helplessness and wanted to visit. Mara conveyed messages of well-wishes to her mother from family and friends everywhere including those from Grenada, Trinidad, England, Spain, Texas, California, Florida, Georgia, New York, New Jersey,

Pennsylvania, Delaware and of course all the local ones in the Washington DC metropolitan area.

Her friend Avis from New York was determined to visit her and so she did. Avis and Denise had developed a friendship seven years prior when they met at the airport on the way to Grenada. Avis had lost her mom and was traveling to Grenada for the burial when there was an overnight delay with their flight. They decided to share a hotel room and had remained friends since. When they got to Grenada, Denise had encouraged her younger sister, Yvonne, to attend Avis' mother's funeral with her. Another friend, Marge, in Marietta, Georgia as well as Marge's daughter Amicah and Amicah's son Miguel also traveled to Maryland to visit Denise. Everyone who visited, complimented Denise on her progress and prayed for her full recovery. Although she was not able to communicate with her visitors in ways that they were able to understand, they were convinced that she felt their presence, heard their prayers, and prayed herself. Her faith was always important to her. They played music for her, selecting songs that they knew she would recognize. Avis smiled when she thought that Denise moved her right leg in response to the music. Her faith reassured her, she said, that Denise would recover.

As the days on dialysis progressed, Mara noticed drastic improvements in her mother's condition. Some of the swelling went down.

Denise's other close friends Lori, Breana, Cathy, Myrna, and Hope were present quite often to cheer Denise on and to support her daughter. During this time, the physicians were concerned about Denise being exposed to anything that could cause more infections as they were already treating her for infections. With that in mind, Mara broached the subject with Dr. Miles who suggested that limiting visitors or preventing visits from those with a cold or flu-like symptoms, would be best for her recovery. Mara sent out a group text:

Hello everyone, please remember that mummy is still critically ill. Please feel free to visit her in the ICU at Northern Metropolitan Hospital and pray with her. She does not need anything in her room—no flowers, no plants, no food, or fruits. If you have a cold or signs of it, please postpone your visit for a later date when all signs of the cold are gone. There are gloves in the room that the nurses may ask you to wear. Thanks for the continued prayers and support.

There was one male dialysis nurse, Alvin, who talked to Mara about his family while he provided dialysis. He also talked about Denise's progress.

"I think your mother is doing well," he said. "Don't you see the changes? I notice changes. She is looking around. She moves her right leg."

Mara smiled, "Yes but the intensivist told me that's what I want to see."

Alvin turned to look at Mara and raised his eyebrows as if he were surprised. They continued to speak about their jobs. He asked Mara for her business card. Was that a frown on her mother's face? Her eyes were closed, but Mara could swear that was a frown. Was she imagining it? She leaned forward, watching her mother closely, a small smile on her lips. Alvin said, "Ms. Mitchell, it's only for business, only for business." Mara laughed. "Oh, you saw it too?" He smiled, nodded. "I told you she's improving."

Alvin told Mara, out of earshot of Denise, that she would need to transfer to a long-term acute care hospital (LTACH). He knew other dialysis nurses who worked at a few of the LTACHs, he said, and could get their feedback if she would like. Mara had not been to any of the LTACHs. She said she would appreciate any information that she received about them.

***

Since the day after the exchange of cards with Alvin, Mara could see that whenever that dialysis nurse entered Denise's room, whether it was for dialysis or just a quick visit to check on her, her eyebrows would furrow, and she did not seem happy. Mara would smile, though, because to her it meant that her mother was as present and as involved as ever. She had an opinion, and she would let her know it.

104

Chapter 12

Anxiety and uninformed care

The surgeon at Northern Metropolitan Hospital, Dr. Sam, did the second part of the surgery that he had planned from the beginning—the stent placement. It went well.

Denise remained on the ventilator. She was following commands to some extent; she wiggled her toes, squeezed with her right hand. That was all she could do with the right hand, and she tracked with her eyes. She was unable to move her left arm or hand. Mara asked Dr. Miles over the phone, to place an order to have the physical and occupational therapists work with her mother to address her inability to move her left arm. Mara also told her about the concern for the possible development of foot drop, a condition that would prevent Denise from being able to lift the front part of her foot and could also cause heel ulcers. Dr. Miles acknowledged the request from Mara with 'okay.' It was a brief conversation when Mara had called for an update. The therapists did not work with Denise. They provided a splint for the left hand

and a boot to help to prevent foot drop. The therapists made a schedule for the splint and one for the boot. They posted the schedules on the wall, over Denise's bed.

As a result of the strokes, Denise was now unable to turn herself in the bed, so she relied on the staff to turn her frequently. Despite the frequent turning, there were signs of early skin breakdown. The nurses told Mara they were turning her every two hours. She wondered whether this was so. Were they only doing things like that when people were around? That, she felt, she had to leave up to the staff's conscience. There was no way of knowing. Unfortunately, it was Denise's skin to suffer the consequences and provide answers. Breana, with her nursing experience and her knowledge of the system, requested a special mattress to prevent further skin breakdown. The mattress was provided, and a special cream was ordered by Dr. Miles to place on the affected area.

There was not much opportunity for the therapists to work with Denise as she was too sedated and unable to participate. Once she grimaced, the nurses medicated her for pain with dilaudid and fentanyl. In addition, the staff assessed that she exhibited signs of anxiety, so she was medicated with seroquel. Her body's ability to rid itself of all of these medications would more than likely be significantly slower than that of another person who was not experiencing renal impairment, as well as all of the other complications.

Noting all of this, Mara began to express her concern about the narcotics and her mother's sluggish responses. Was she being a constant bother to the nurses? But it is not their mother! If I do not advocate for her, who will? All aspects of her mother's care were extremely important to Mara. Her constant presence at her mother's bedside was because she wanted to support her mother's recovery from head to toe. She hoped the staff realized that and that she was not visiting because she wanted to critique. Still, she could not bother too much about that. She had enough to worry about. Her observations were about everything, and not focused on one area or system.

Care continued at the Northern Metropolitan Hospital. *But you need to let the patient know!* It was a refrain that kept echoing in her mind as she sat at her mother's bedside and saw the way that the staff, nurses, and respiratory therapists alike, started to suction her mother's tracheostomy or perform other tasks without informing her ahead of time. Was it just her training? Wasn't it the same training they received? Wouldn't anyone know that the sudden interruption to rest would frighten a patient?

Mara started to make suggestions that they inform her mother prior to providing care. They ignored her. Without wanting to overstep her boundaries, she started to ask the staff about their intentions as they entered the room. One nurse, Jasmine, walked into the room.

"Hi. What are you going to do?" Mara asked, forcing Jasmine to halt mid-stride before reaching the bed.

"I have to flush the feeding tube and hang a new bag of formula."

Jasmine smiled and continued to walk closer to the bed. Relieved, Mara smiled in kind, then promptly relayed the information to her mother.

"Mummy your nurse is going to flush the tube in your stomach, okay? Then you will have more feeding."

Denise opened her right eye and closed it again. The nurse proceeded with using a syringe to flush water through the tube and hung the bag as she said, but still did not say anything to Denise.

There were other days, when Mara received some questioning and disapproving expressions from the staff when she asked about their intentions as they entered the room, but Mara continued to do so anyway. If they chose not to inform their patient, then she would. There was no way to control this pattern while she was at work or when she stepped away from her mother's bedside. She hoped that at some point they would realize that it was a real person in the bed to whom they were providing care. The fact that Denise was not able to communicate with them and was on the ventilator, did not suggest that there was a problem with her hearing. She was also able to feel both physically and emotionally. The nurses were always very polite, but just not willing to deviate from their norm. And that, Mara thought, was the reason they labeled her mother as having anxiety. Of course, she was anxious! Who wouldn't be, feeling these frequent movements and not understanding them or knowing when to expect them?

When the nurses started to medicate Denise for anxiety, Mara decided to talk to the charge nurse. Charge nurse Amy was very friendly and readily available. She reassured Mara that she would address her concerns with the staff. Mara did not know if the response she received was to appease her or if it was sincere. She chose to believe the latter. She continued to request prayers from her mother's friends and family.

***

A couple more days passed. The staff continued to be very polite to the daughter; however, nothing changed regarding the provision of care to her mother. Was their maxim: *ignore them even as you are killing them with kindness?* She spoke with the attending physician Dr. Thompson when he walked into her mother's room. Mara was sitting on the chair next to her mother.

"My mom is unable to participate in her care because she is being kept in a sedated state. Can you please discontinue the order for the narcotics and anything else that may be contributing to that?"

"Sure, let's see how she does without sedation," the physician said, as he walked over to Denise. She was able to look up at the physician with her right eye partially open. He examined her, then started walking out of the room. As a second thought, Dr. Thompson said, "Enjoy your visit."

The physician discontinued the order for the narcotics. Her mother was now more alert. She was not receiving therapy because the staff did not think that she would participate, even though she was more awake. A day after the physician discontinued the narcotics, the social worker called Mara. She wanted to discuss discharge plans.

Chapter 13

Discharge planning

While Mara did not have the expectation that her mother would stay at the hospital indefinitely, she was also not expecting her to be discharged without having an opportunity to make more progress. Was that how this hospital operated? Did they think she was asking too many questions? If they were no longer giving her narcotics, did they feel their job was done? After the aortic dissection and stroke in 2010, Denise had received physical, occupational, and speech therapy—and she had managed to return to her baseline. In 2010, the therapy services were initiated as soon as Denise became alert, even while she remained on the ventilator. Mara thought with longing of the treatment at University Hospital in 2010. In her present condition at the Northern Metropolitan Hospital, the discharge plan was to transfer her without having received therapy services and of course no plan for those services to continue at a long-term acute care hospital, according to the social worker.

February 4, 2017

To: Physician Advisor/Administration at Northern Metropolitan Hospital

I am writing to you regarding my mother, Denise Mitchell who has been a patient at Northern Metropolitan Hospital since November 25, 2016. The staff has been wonderful and very responsive to her needs and in answering my questions. I am happy that she is in such a reputable hospital; however, I have some concerns which I am confident you will be able to help me address.

Surgery was performed for a descending aortic dissection on 12/7/16. Unfortunately, since the surgery, she has experienced a number of setbacks. These setbacks include strokes of which I was not made aware of initially and that is concerning. I understand that the more recent CT scan shows subarachnoid hemorrhage. The other issue is that after she was extubated and received Losartan on 12/9/16, it became apparent that she may have had a reaction to this medication, in addition to having heparin induced thrombocytopenia. This required her to be reintubated and she has been back on the ventilator since 12/9/16. Unfortunately, she received Losartan a second time which compounded the first reaction of angioedema. She then received Lisinopril even after the swelling was still there from two exposures.

She is not receiving physical therapy because she has been too sedated to participate. After the propofol was turned off, she was then medicated with dilaudid and seroquel. She has received several doses of narcotics that kept her in a constant sleepy state and have prevented her from waking up fully to participate in her care. I have witnessed staff begin to suction or perform tasks without informing her of what is about to be done. She is unable to communicate and may possibly be afraid. Instead of being reassured that she is safe and okay, she was being medicated for agitation. This seems to be a vicious cycle.

She was being treated unnecessarily for hypertension with systolic blood pressure readings over two hundred. The blood pressure measurement was performed with a cuff on her lower extremity. After an arterial line was placed, it was found that there was a 100-point difference from the cuff reading and the A-line. A combination of several doses of narcotics as well as hypertensive medications, I believe have contributed to impaired kidney function. Now, she needs dialysis.

I am being told that she is not tracking, but I have noticed some improvements with her in the past three days. She has been more awake and has followed some commands. Once the narcotics have stopped, she has been able to respond in some way. It is unfortunate that now that she is making some sort of progress, the plan is to discharge her without allowing her more time to make progress. Once the providers give up on their patients who are fighting to stay alive, this lack of hope can be felt by the patients and families and as a result the patients give up as well.

I am confident that we can work together in addressing these concerns, with the hope that my mother can be weaned off the vent prior to discharge from Northern Metropolitan Hospital. Thanks again for your efforts in trying to ensure that my mother gets good medical care.

For a moment, Mara thought about the fact that her letter could result in her being labeled a querulous trouble-maker; however, she knew that she would be the one to accurately label herself as an advocate. It was their choice to think of her in whatever way they chose, but it was not their right to allow harm to be brought to her mother.

Mara assumed that administration would review her mother's chart when they received the letter. There was no reason for her to be anything but humble as she really needed a positive response and was grateful for the progress that her mother had made. Mara received a written response from someone in leadership that same evening. His letter read:

Dear Ms. Mitchell,

Thank you very much for drawing my attention to your mother's situation. I am very sorry about all of the recent events surrounding her hospitalization and will review her case on Monday. As I am not acting as a physician advisor nowadays, I have not been involved in her situation at all but have already forwarded your communication to some of the appropriate members of our team.

Sincerely

A few days later, Mara received a telephone call from one of the individuals to whom her concerns were forwarded, Dr. Hyland. That physician was directly connected to the care management department. This is the department that is responsible for discharge planning for the patients at the hospital. Dr. Hyland told Mara, "The social worker should not have called you to discuss discharge planning. She contacted you prematurely."

Mara gasped. As she listened to Dr. Hyland, Mara silently wondered: *Why does it sound as if she is blaming the social worker? I wrote a detailed letter. What about the medical issues?* The conversation lasted for about five minutes and Dr. Hyland focused on the discharge process and not on any of the medical issues that Mara had mentioned in her letter. The physician told Mara, "When your mother is stable for discharge, she can be transferred to another facility to continue the weaning process from the ventilator."

That evening, when Mara went to visit her mother, she saw Laney, the director of nursing on the unit. The director held a folder up to her chest and had a broad smile on her face. She was wearing a light blue pair of scrubs with a white lab coat over the scrubs. She was a Caucasian woman, in her late fifties. She wore a short haircut, just underneath her earlobes. There were streaks of gray in her brunette hair. She approached Mara at her mother's doorway.

"Hi there, thanks for your letter. I am sorry to hear about the issues with your mom. I will be speaking with the staff this evening," and she nodded her head, in apparent confirmation of her words. Mara smiled in acknowledgement.

"If you'll excuse me," Laney said as she walked toward her office which was two doors away.

Mara went into her mother's room and sat next to her. She gently rested her hand on her mother's hand. She sat in silence for most of the visit. Before she left her mother's bedside that evening, the assigned nurse, April, a dark-skinned petite woman, a couple of inches taller than Mara, placed her hand on Mara's shoulder.

"You wrote a good letter," she said. "It is good to hear what families think."

Apart from the physician who had responded to inform Mara that he had forwarded her email to the correct individual, Mara noted, the responses that she had received were not in writing. As she processed the cautious responses that she had received, she thought that it was obvious that the individuals in leadership were only concerned about protecting themselves and not the helpless patient who was receiving care at their hospital. Nevertheless, they had acknowledged her concerns in some form and were aware that she was concerned and involved in her mother's care.

The following evening, Mara saw the charge nurse, Amy, as well as the intensivist, Dr. Miles, talking in the hallway near to her mother's room. She approached them.

"Hi, excuse me for a minute. I would like to see my mom out of the bed and sitting up in the chair. The fact that she is on the ventilator is not a reason for her to be confined to the bed and develop more infections and pressure ulcers."

The two ladies, both with concerned expressions, looked down at Mara.

"We'll get her out of the bed." Dr. Miles said.

Mara smiled at them and said, "thank you" as she walked away and into her mother's room.

***

On February 10, 2017, the next morning, Mara called her mother's nurse at Northern Metropolitan Hospital. Emily, the nurse, with excitement in her voice said, "your mom was placed in the chair a few minutes ago!" Mara smiled, "Oh, that is great! I am so happy to hear that. How is she doing?" She heard rustling sounds of paper from Emily's end.

"Um...she is stable. She does not seem to be in any type of distress. Her vitals and labs are okay," Emily said, but it sounded to Mara as though she was slightly distracted.

Still smiling, Mara said, "okay, thanks Emily. I will see her this evening after work." Emily immediately responded, "okay sure. See you later."

In the evening, when Mara arrived at her mother's room, Emily walked into the room shortly after. She smiled at Mara. "Hi! Your mom did not seem to be comfortable in the chair earlier today, so after about ten minutes, we brought her back to the bed," she said.

Mara raised her eyebrows and turned her head to the side.

"Well, which is understandable. She had been bedbound for almost two months. She needs more time to be able to tolerate sitting up for longer periods."

"Yes, you're right," Emily said, only half smiling now.

Mara thought, though, that if they continued to transfer Denise to the chair, at least once per day, she would be able to tolerate sitting up for longer periods as time passed.

Mara continued to visit with her mother that evening. She pulled the chair a little closer to her mother's bed. Emily walked in with another young lady, who was a few inches taller than her and was walking very slowly. The other lady had both of her hands in the front pockets of the scrubs that she was wearing.

"This is Kymberly. She will be your mom's night nurse," Emily said.

"Hi Kymberly. I am Mara," she said with a smile. Kymberly flashed a quick smile then immediately afterward, assumed a serious expression.

Emily said, "okay… I left an extra bag of IV fluid there because this one will finish in an hour." They walked over to Denise. Kymberly leaned over a bit closer to her, with one hand on the siderail and introduced herself, "Ms. Mitchell. My name is Kymberly. I will be your nurse tonight."

Denise opened her right eye and looked up at Kymberly. The nurses did not say anything else. They both turned and walked out of the room. About half hour later, Kymberly and one of the nursing assistants entered the room with towels and washcloths in their hands. Kymberly smiled as she got closer to Mara and as she placed the linen on the bed.

"Will you excuse us? We need to change her."

Mara stood up from the chair, "Sure. I just need to see her back when you turn her." Kymberly walked over to the other side of the bed, away from the side that Mara was standing. "

Okay, we can turn her," she said. They kept the head of the bed at about a forty-five-degree angle. The nursing assistant pulled the sheet on the bed, closer to herself and she then used it to help support Denise to turn on her right side. Kymberly supported Denise's back with her hands when they turned her toward Kymberly. Mara took a mental note: *Okay. The excoriation on her lower back is healing. Good.* She said to Kymberly and the nursing assistant, "Thanks. I will wait outside the room." She stepped out of the room and within five minutes, she heard: "Ms. Mitchell! Ms. Mitchell!" She immediately walked back to the door and saw her mother lying flat on the bed while her nurse performed chest compressions.

Naturally, she attempted to enter the room, but Kymberly shouted, "Please step out!" Mara stood near the doorway of her mother's room. She started to tremble with fear of what was happening to her mother. An announcement was made on the overhead intercom system for a code and a swarm of hospital personnel rushed into the room. A few minutes later, Dr. Miles approached Mara, "Your mom is okay. We have not figured out what caused her to become unresponsive. Any thoughts on changing her from full code to do not resuscitate?"

Mara's arms were folded as she leaned against the wall outside of her mother's room. She said calmly, "No. She'll remain full code."

At a moment like this, is that what she should be asking?! Mara wanted to know what had caused her mother to become unresponsive.

She called her mother's friend Breana, "The nurse and nursing assistant went to change mummy and they lowered the head of the bed. She became unconscious for a few minutes, and they called a code. The intensivist said that she is okay now. I'm still waiting outside because they're still attending to her."

Breana sounded concerned. "Really? It could be because of fluid shift, if the head of the bed was lowered abruptly. Do you need me to come?"

Mara replied, "No. They said she is okay right now, so I am okay. Thanks."

They ended their call shortly after that. A few minutes later, Denise's friend Ali called Mara to check on Denise's status. Mara described her mother's unresponsiveness the same way she had described it to Breana. Aunt Ali replied, "Oh. It was probably a mucus plug."

Mara accepted both responses as possibilities. When Mara walked back into the room, she said to Kymberly who was cleaning the bedside table.

"I realized that my mom became unresponsive after the head of the bed was lowered. The head of the bed should be lowered gradually next time because it could be fluid shift or perhaps a mucus plug.

Kymberly continued to focus on the bedside table but nodded, "Okay, sure."

Mara did not know this about the lowering of the head of the bed to be a fact in this case, however, it was worth a try. Were they listening? Were they annoyed? Would they try to find out what was going on? What would they do? If she, a professional, felt like this, what did family members who had no information about nursing or medical care feel in these situations?

On February 14, 2017, there was a repeat of this scenario just a few short days later. Denise once again became unresponsive, and Mara noticed that it happened when the head of the bed was lowered during personal care. It appears everything negative at that place, had to occur at least twice.

The question about code status had been raised by Dr. Miles to Mara, after Denise's first incident of loss of consciousness. Denise was a full code; if her heart stopped, they were to do everything to save her. The intensivist initiated that discussion again, Mara thought, as a broken record.

Mara was not making any changes with that plan. She said slowly, deliberately, "My 61-year-old mother walked into the emergency room with complaints of back pain. She has had a number of setbacks, no fault of hers and you are quick to give up on her."

The intensivist did not stop there. She contacted Mara's aunt Simone, Denise's sister who was an emergency room physician in Grenada and tried to convince her that Denise's recovery was hopeless. No. Mara thought, we will stay the course. She remembered that her mother used to make fun of her whenever she used that phrase but this time, she felt, it was most appropriate. We will stay the course.

While Mara was telling herself that she was determined to allow her mother to die with dignity when and if the time came, a segment on aortic dissection was aired on one of the local television networks. It was about the Northern Metropolitan Hospital. She saw the segment on her television, on the same evening that she met Dr. Miles at her mother's bedside. The documentary advertised the hospital's expertise in caring for patients with aortic dissection. Mara believed that medical errors could occur at any hospital or facility; however, how the issues are addressed would make a difference. If the doctors or nurses recognized or were made aware that there was a drastic change with their patient's condition, it would be their duty to correct the problems, not cover-up. Mara thought that they should have transferred Denise out of their care when it became too complex for them to continue to care for her. If that was what they were feeling, however expert they might feel they were, they should admit that they were out of ideas in this situation and recommend that her care be turned over to another facility.

***

On February 18, 2017, Denise was making slow progress. Nonetheless, it was progress. The staff continued to transfer her to the chair. Each day she tolerated sitting up for a longer period than the previous day. As Dr. Miles walked by Denise's room; she saw Mara sitting in the room next to Denise's bed. Dr. Miles smiled. She walked to the doorway, paused, and then walked further into the room. She updated Mara as she nodded her head with each sentence, "Your mom, I have seen her sitting in the chair. She seems comfortable. She withdraws better when pain or pressure is applied. She localizes pain. She tracks a little with her eyes during assessments. She squeezes with her right hand and wiggles her toes."

Those were not observations that Mara had expected the intensivist to ever acknowledge.

"Yes, she's a fighter," Mara said, happy Dr. Miles, finally realized what she already knew.

"Good. Okay, take care." Dr. Miles exited the room.

As the days passed, Mara began to feel that her mom was now approaching discharge but required a few revisions with the feeding tube. The feeding tube needed to be flushed manually with water before and after her medications and feeding; however, there were complications. The tube clogged a couple of times and was also dislodged. The interventional radiologist replaced it with a new tube which seemed to function well.

Chapter 14

Plan to transfer to long-term acute care hospital

Denise needed to be transferred to a long-term acute care hospital, where she would continue to be weaned from the ventilator, have dialysis and, at her daughter's request, receive therapy services. This was even though she was not receiving therapy at the Northern Metropolitan Hospital. There were a few factors to be considered when selecting a facility.

In the Washington DC metropolitan area, there were not many choices of vent-weaning facilities from which her family could select. Only those that were in network with her health insurance could be considered. Proximity to her home or her daughter's home was important. Not all vent-weaning facilities provided dialysis. The list was quite short. Mara got assistance from her aunts, her mother's friends who researched the facilities to make the best decision on the facility choice to meet Denise's needs. The closest facility was unable to accept her because they thought that she was too complex, and they would not be able to address her needs. Mara appreciated the honesty.

The next close facility felt the same way but simply said that they could not accept her. Her mother required more care than they could provide but they eventually responded after the social worker sent a second request and said that they did not have any beds available. It also did not help that the physicians had documented that Denise had a poor prognosis and had never updated their documentation to indicate the progress that she had made. They omitted the documentation that would have indicated that it was the care that she received from their hospital that resulted in her poor prognosis.

Finally, she was accepted at a facility in Baltimore. It was more than fifty-four miles away from Mara's home and workplace. She did not have a choice. In rush hour traffic, this would be an hour and ten minutes away. At first, Mara was concerned about the distance, but she was also concerned and interested to know that the facility was equipped and appropriate to care for her mother.

On February 22, 2017, a few days before her mother was scheduled to transfer to the long-term acute care hospital, Mara received a telephone call from Maribeth, the admission's nurse liaison.

"Your mother would receive dialysis, physical, occupational, speech and respiratory therapy services at the facility," Maribeth explained. "There are doctors on site around the clock. The success rate of weaning is greater than eighty five percent. The unit where your mother would be placed is like a mini-intensive care unit. There are about twenty-five patients total on the unit. Your mother would need to have a telemetry bed, where she would be monitored closely. There is also a wound care team on the unit. The average stay for patients is two to three weeks. Initially, the insurance would authorize a certain number of days and they would need to continue to receive clinical updates from the facility, to continue to approve additional days. In your mom's case, the insurance company approved the first ten days, and no copay is involved. The facility is affiliated with Simion Hospital which is directly across the street. Your mother would have a roommate. Visiting hours are 11am to 8pm, but they are lenient toward individuals who visit late."

Maribeth continued by providing Mara with the address to the facility, phone numbers to the nursing station and pod table, as well as the name of the nurse manager on the unit. Mara received extremely useful information. She was concerned that her mother was being placed so far away but having this much information would be immensely helpful and allay some of her fears.

Mara thought about the information that Maribeth had given her. She was pleased to hear that her mother would receive therapy services. She was even more pleased to learn that there would be doctors around the clock at the facility. Maribeth mentioned that her mother would be monitored closely, and she certainly needed that. The success rate was good, and she expected her mother to be included in that group. Her mother had started to have skin breakdown at the Northern Metropolitan Hospital and that seemed to be under control, but she would benefit from having access to a wound care team as she continued to spend most of her time in the bed. The facility was a long-term acute care hospital, and she was surprised to hear that the average length of stay was two to three weeks. Then why call it long-term? Wouldn't patients expect to have longer stays at long term acute care hospitals? She knew that every patient's experience was different, and she expected that the staff would provide care based on her mother's needs, not on a timeline that was set for everyone. She expected individualized care. Should she ask? Should she not ask? She decided that she would wait and see.

On the day that the hospital scheduled Denise's transfer, there was another problem with the feeding tube in her stomach. The nurse was unable to flush water through it. It was clogged. The social worker rescheduled transportation for the following day to allow time for the nurses to unclog the tube.

Chapter 15

Transfer to Baltimore Long Term Acute Care Hospital

On February 24, 2017, the evening of the actual transfer, Denise's friend, Hope, was at her bedside. She prayed for Denise and reassured her that she would be okay. Myrna planned to drive, so she and Mara met at the Northern Metropolitan Hospital. The staff visited Denise's room to bid farewell and extend well-wishes. Mara was grateful for all that they had done to help to keep her mother alive.

It was now dark. The ambulance crew arrived. The social worker scheduled the ambulance to pick up Denise at 6pm but it was almost 7:30pm when they arrived on the unit. They waited for Denise's nurse and got report from her. They transferred Denise's monitoring and ventilator to their monitor and ventilator. Aunt Myrna and Mara were headed to Baltimore. They followed the ambulance to the facility. It was a long, quiet drive. They could see the paramedic in the back with Denise move around but could not see exactly what she was doing. They just hoped that there was no problem and that whatever she was doing was routine. Finally, after driving for what seemed like an eternity, the ambulance drove onto a property that was private and after looking around for signs, they finally saw the name, Baltimore Long Term Acute Care Hospital. They parked and walked to the entrance.

The security guard at the desk did not seem at all pleased that they had decided to accompany their family member.

"Can I help you?" he said to them. "we're here with Denise Mitchell," Myrna responded. "She just arrived."

The security guard had a serious expression on his face and said, "the facility is very strict with visiting hours which ended at 8pm."

It was approaching 9:30pm. It was not until much later that Mara recalled Maribeth had told her that the facility was lenient with their visiting hours. Someone's information needed to be updated, either Maribeth's or the security guard's. It was important that the information that they communicated to visitors was consistent.

As they walked on to the unit, they met Joe, the physician assistant on duty. He was Caucasian, about six feet two inches tall, average build and he had a smile that made them feel welcomed. That was exactly what they needed. He greeted them and asked, "You're here with…?"

They both responded, "Mitchell."

He introduced himself and said, "Oh yes, you must be her daughter. I heard about you." Mara thought to herself, he has. She wondered what he had heard about her. If she had not felt exhausted, she would have asked. At that point she just wanted to see her mother.

She was curious to know what had been happening in the ambulance. They entered the very warm room. Denise's bed was closer to the window. Her roommate was an older lady who was also on the ventilator. The roommate must have had lots of family and friends or must have been at the facility or away from her home for quite some time. There were greeting cards on the entire wall on her side of the room.

Denise's nurse was Jenny, a very pleasant nurse whose facial appearance, slight build, skin tone and accent told Mara that she must be from the Philippines. Jenny oriented them to the room and to the unit. With a smile on her face, Jenny said, "This is the call bell. If she needs anything, you can press the red button. You can use the call bell also to turn the lights off and on. This door is to the restroom," she said, pointing toward a door at the corner, on the right of Denise's bed. "But since they're both staying in their beds, they won't be using it."

Jenny was smiling throughout and chuckled a little when she said, "do not worry. She is safe." Noting Jenny's attitude toward her mother, Mara could not imagine otherwise.

As she and her Aunt Myrna stood at Denise's bedside, Mara held up a neck roll that Aunt Breana had made for Denise and she said, "Mummy, take this." It was an indescribable feeling when her mother did something that she had not done in a couple of months. She reached with her right hand, took the neck roll from her daughter, and just held on to it. Mara and her aunt Myrna looked at each other in amazement. A little more than two months prior, Denise had not been able to move any of her extremities. Now, she raised her arm up and very naturally took this neck roll and kept holding it. Myrna and Mara, standing at the bedside, chuckled with excitement. Denise looked at them a bit questioningly, they thought, but she was unable to speak since she was still on the vent. They could only imagine the questions that were on her mind. They complimented her on her progress. Denise seemed to be a bit uncomfortable, and they attributed her discomfort to the temperature in the room. It was extremely warm. At least they were able to express themselves, but she was not able to do the same.

Mara asked Jenny, "Can she have a fan in here?" Jenny turned away from the computer in the room to face Mara and said, "Oh yes. You can bring one in, and it would need to be approved by the engineering department." Both Myrna and Mara said, "okay, thank you." Jenny closed the screen on the computer and said, "Okay, I will be out there. Call if you need anything." Myrna and Mara both smiled at Jenny and said, "Thanks again. We are leaving now." It was approaching 11:30pm. They wished Denise a good night. Her eyes looked sad, as if she did not want them to leave. Mara promised to see her the next day. Well, she thought, that was if the security guard did not prohibit them from returning to the facility. They were visiting extremely late.

The next morning, Mara called the unit at the facility where her mother was located. She asked to speak with the nurse who was caring for her mother. A lady named Dana came on the line and introduced herself as Denise's nurse. Mara identified herself and asked for an update on her mother; how she had spent the night, how she was responding, and what the plans were for her that day. Dana was very direct. She provided Mara with an update as if she were giving report to one of her colleagues. That was not an issue at all. In fact, Mara really appreciated her diligence. She told Mara that her mother was not responding to commands. She had gotten report from the previous nurse that Denise had not slept during the night and that the physical and occupational therapists were scheduled to perform an evaluation that day. The transition from the acute care hospital to the long-term acute care hospital seemed to have caused some sort of setback for Denise. She was not responding to commands because she had not slept the previous night and she had not slept that night because she was confused and did not know where she was; Myrna and Mara had told her, but she was confused. In addition, the room was extremely warm. Her brain had been through so much that she required more time to process things. Patience, Mara thought, was a virtue, and now a necessity from everyone involved.

After her workday ended, Mara drove an hour and ten minutes, eager to see her mother. Denise was very drowsy. She recognized her daughter but was not responding as she had done prior to leaving the Northern Metropolitan Hospital or even the night that she arrived at this facility. Mara met the nurse, Dana, whom she had spoken with earlier that day. Dana had a serious expression but answered all of Mara's questions. She updated her on the events of the day. She folded her arms as she spoke.

"The therapists came to see her today, but they were not able to work with her because she was very sleepy."

Mara continuing to be attentive to her mother, gently stroked her left arm. "Okay, thanks" she said.

Dana tidied the bedside table and walked out of the room. As Dana's shift ended, she walked into the room with Ann, the oncoming nurse for the night shift. Dana introduced Ann to Denise and to Mara. They performed bedside report as Dana provided Ann with pertinent information regarding Denise's status and care. They looked at all the tubes and lines: the gastrostomy-jejunostomy or feeding tube, dialysis catheter, peripherally inserted central line (PICC line), foley catheter and rectal tube. They also looked...or, more accurately, glanced quickly...at the settings on the ventilator. They turned Denise to her side and they examined the excoriation on her lower back. Everything was okay from the nurse's report.

A few minutes after the nurses left the room, two respiratory therapists walked into the room: Gail, who was leaving for the evening and Greg, who was the night respiratory therapist. They introduced themselves to their patient and to her daughter. They walked over to the ventilator and looked at the settings. The respiratory therapists placed Denise on full ventilator support when she arrived at the facility. At the Northern Metropolitan Hospital, she had been on CPAP mode which required her to do some of the work of breathing with some assistance from the vent. Here, she had started the process all over, it seemed. Mara inquired from the therapists about the plan and informed them that her mother had been on CPAP setting on the ventilator at the other hospital and that she was surprised to see that she was on full vent support. Gail raised her eyebrows, as though surprised to learn about Denise being on CPAP previously.

"Really?" she said. "We have not received documentation from the Northern Metropolitan Hospital on your mom's progress with the vent. We assumed that she was on full ventilator support, and we would be the first to start the weaning process."

To Mara, this was very disappointing to hear. So, the hospitals had not been in communication about a patient they transferred? The therapists continued their report with each other and then walked out of the room. Mara spent another hour at her mother's bedside. There was an announcement on the intercom system, that visiting hours would end in fifteen minutes. At that time, Mara said a prayer at her mother's bedside. She kissed and hugged her goodnight and walked out of the room. Her mother's nurse and other staff were sitting outside of her room at the pod table. She said to them, "have a goodnight. Please call me if there are any issues during the night." One of the ladies at the desk smiled at Mara and said, "Do not worry. There will not be any issues." Mara continued to walk toward the exit for the unit. As she got to the front desk, she noticed that the security guard from the previous night was not there. Instead, it was a very friendly lady who, Mara realized had made the announcement about visiting hours. This lady, although she had just made the announcement, seemed to want visitors to stay or to chat with her because she started a conversation with Mara about her day and said that her shift would end in another couple of hours. They talked for a few minutes and then they wished each other a goodnight and Mara left. So, whatever the policy might be, individuals made a difference.

The next morning, Mara contacted the social worker at the Northern Metropolitan Hospital and requested that she send her mother's respiratory therapy's progress notes to the Baltimore Long Term Acute Care Hospital. Those notes would be among the most significant information related to Denise's care. She had been transferred there to be weaned off the ventilator. It did not make sense that the discharge planner omitted the respiratory therapy's notes from the discharge packet or from the information that that person sent to them electronically. She was troubled that while information about her—the daughter, had preceded Denise to the facility, the patient-related information had not made it on time. Mara thought, it was just an oversight. She followed up with the facility in Baltimore and learned that the physician had been given the newly sent documentation. She spoke with her mother's nurse Karen over the phone.

"We don't all have access to all of the patient's information," Karen informed Mara. According to Karen, "the physician decides what would be shared with the staff."

Their process was different from what Mara was used to. Now, her mother's ventilator weaning process depended, she felt, on whether the physician wanted to share the information that he received with the respiratory therapists. She did not want to seem unreasonable, but her mother was there for health care reasons, and one always had to be thinking of the insurance—of how much time would be allowed at the facility.

After work, Mara visited her mother. Denise remained on full ventilator support. She was very drowsy. She opened her eyes and looked at her daughter but did not respond to commands. Her heart rate was extremely fast. She was on telemetry monitoring and so depending on the settings on the monitor, the alarms were triggered frequently. Her nurse entered the room a few times, looked at her and the monitor and pressed the silence button.

The family for the patient in the first bed was visiting that evening—the patient's husband and daughter. They dressed themselves in the isolation gowns and entered the room. Watching, Mara reflected that she had thought her mother was no longer on isolation because the providers did not mention it when she was leaving the Northern Metropolitan Hospital and the staff was not wearing the isolation gown when they cared for her mother at this new facility. Her concern now was that her mother had been placed in an isolation room with another patient who had some sort of infection. The night nurse walked into the room and Mara inquired from her about her mother's status. Was she on isolation? The nurse informed her that the report she had been given was that her mother was on isolation and that there was a sign on the door. Mara walked back to the door and realized that there was indeed a sign, but it was at the top of the door—not very noticeable and no one had pointed it out until that moment. Shouldn't caregivers be forthcoming with pertinent information related to her mother? She donned the gown and chose not to make an issue out of this matter. There was more at stake here.

Meanwhile, Denise was on and off with antibiotics. She was kept on isolation at the facility.

At times, when Mara was at her mother's bedside, the nurses reported to each other that she had an infection, and at other times, in their bedside report, they would say that she had an infection in the past.

Chapter 16

Progress

The next day, the phone call to the nurse for update provided information that was a bit more promising. Although the chest x-ray indicated that Denise had pneumonia again, despite being weak she was consistently following commands. This was an improvement. The news pleased Mara. The doctors ordered intravenous fluids and antibiotics for Denise. Her vital signs were fluctuating, and she had been medicated by the nurse for high blood pressure at least once during that day, in addition to being given her routine blood pressure medications.

The visit to her mother in the evening was a little more satisfying than had been previous days' visits for Mara. Now, Denise was smiling. She kept her eyes on her daughter throughout the evening. Whenever Mara changed positions or moved from one side of the bed to the other, her mother followed her with her eyes. When Mara noticed that was happening, she moved more often so she could get a response from her mother. She was overly excited to observe the progress that her mother had made. Then came the announcement that visiting hours had ended. Mara said a prayer at her mother's bedside and left.

To friends and family, she continued to send text messages with updates, always including a request for prayers.

On the following morning, the report from the nurse was about the same as the previous day's report. Denise was following commands. When Mara saw her that evening, Denise smiled more and continued to follow commands. However, there were moments that she seemed uncertain as to whether she was responding appropriately. She turned her head to look at her right foot to see if she had moved it. This was major improvement from the weeks that she had seen her mother at the Northern Metropolitan Hospital, when all she did at first was blink, then later opened her eyes fully. Mara had not wanted those days at the Northern Metropolitan Hospital to be her mother's last moments. No one who cared about her wanted her to just lay there and not be able to communicate, especially knowing the circumstances that had contributed to her current condition.

Denise continued to make progress, every day. To remind Denise to use her extremities and to try to participate in her care, Mara applied lip gloss to her mother's lips. She continued to do so for a couple of days, until Denise realized that she should fold her lips and help to moisten the top lip with the bottom and vice versa. As the days passed, Mara handed her mother the lip gloss and Denise applied it herself. Progress! This did not seem to be as exciting for Denise as it was for Mara. It was ninety-five days since she walked into the emergency room at Northern Metropolitan Hospital. Denise was unaware of the amount of time that had passed or the extent of changes to her condition and so she showed no enthusiasm about the simple things that gave her daughter joy. Mara was extremely excited to see her mother apply lip gloss. Mara recorded Denise's movements as she applied lip gloss. Denise simply stared at her, wondering why her daughter looked at her so intently.

Mara decided to help her mother advance to other tasks. The room was very warm, and although Mara and later Denise's friend Andrina brought a replacement desk fan to the room, the staff did not always turn it on for several reasons. She handed her mother a hand-held fan that she received from her friend Candy and Denise proceeded to fan herself. Again, this was exciting to witness. Mara laughed aloud, then smiled as her mother responded with a smile. To those who paid attention to detail, the minute changes in her condition were very noticeable. Mara performed passive range of motion exercises. She exercised her mother's limbs by holding her foot gently in her hand and moving it. She did the same with her mother's arms and eventually Denise participated. Mara applied lotion to her mother's arms and legs every evening. She asked her to lift her right arm and both of her legs as many as ten times each or until Denise was unable to perform due to exhaustion. Initially, those exercises were done as Mara supported Denise's elbows or knees, depending on what was being exercised. Later, Denise was able to perform the exercises without requiring much support.

***

As the days progressed, Denise became more alert at the long-term acute care hospital. She was not actually receiving therapy. She was placed in a program that the physiatrist oversaw. The facility referred to the program as a coma program. The program was geared toward assisting patients to become more alert and responsive. The therapists worked with Denise at the bedside. They gave her exercises to help her to become more aware of her surroundings. The therapists asked her to identify family members from photos that Mara had provided per their request. They asked her to identify objects, to be able to respond appropriately 'yes' or 'no' to various questions and to be able to express her needs. They were helpful exercises, her daughter thought. Mara appreciated the program but, as the days passed, she thought that the fact that her mother remained in the bed without being involved in active therapy was not sufficient. She requested that the therapists be more active with her mother. She stressed the need for Denise to be out of the bed and sitting in the chair for several reasons.

It was unfortunate, she thought now, that once again, the family needed to make suggestions with regards to the provision of health care for positive outcomes. Denise had been on the ventilator for three months. Being in an upright position in the chair frequently would help to expand her lungs. It would help to relieve pressure on her back and help to prevent pressure ulcers. It would help her to become stronger and be able to participate in her care. Mara told the therapists that prior to her arrival at the facility, her mother had been accustomed to sitting in the chair even if it was for short periods. She expressed her concern that her mother's care in certain areas was not going in the direction that she had expected. There was no explanation as to why, shortly after Denise transferred to the facility, she had been less alert and less responsive than she had been just prior to her transfer. Mara asked questions and based on responses, speculated about why this might be. She wondered now about information shared between facilities. The facility here did not seem aware that Denise had already been sitting upright in the chair prior to the transfer.

Thinking about her own training, she reflected that communication or lack of communication especially in the setting of patient care can prove to be detrimental to patients. On the other hand, she reflected, a business-minded individual who would not accept the health care system as a service for the betterment of health would have a different focus. That individual may be able to recognize communication or lack of communication in a patient-related setting as having a positive or negative impact on factors such as time and financial resources. It may be time-consuming to provide appropriate care and communicate the patient's needs to those who would need all the pertinent information to continue to provide proper care. It may also require the use of more resources to ensure that all needs are met but as Mara considered those factors, her mother's recovery and her life significantly outweighed those factors. Was she seeing the health service differently because of her close personal interests now? She thought about critiques she had in the past but had not voiced. But there were attitudes that she felt sure she had not. ...and was not seeing...every day around her. She really had to think about this. But there were good facilities. University Hospital proved that. Yes. There were good ones, with both administration and workers playing their part. So, there were distinct cultures of care operating in different places. Even within one facility, there could be various levels of care depending on the attitude and interest of a specific caregiver. She continued to see her mother daily and she remained informed about her status. She asked about her vital signs, lab results and any other notable changes. There was some resistance from a few of the nurses, but for the most part they provided her with the information that she requested. Asking the nurses about her mother's laboratory results and vital signs was, she felt, in no way a hindrance to the delivery of care. Her aunts Ali and Simone were quite willing and able to help her interpret those values and make assessments, and they provided solicited opinions and advice. Denise continued dialysis and her kidney function slowly improved. It helped having people who knew the system and the language of medical care.

After a few weeks of her mother being at the long-term acute care hospital, Mara received a phone call from Terri, a social worker. Terri explained that she was helping her coworker. She provided the name and contact information of Denise's assigned social worker as well as of the director of social work. Terri completed an assessment over the phone with Mara. She asked questions about Denise's prior living arrangements—who she lived with, how many steps there were to enter her house and how many steps there were to get to her bedroom, her level of functioning prior to being hospitalized, whether or not she had an

Advanced Directive, whether or not she used assistive devices such as a cane, walker or wheelchair; she wanted to know how she got to medical appointments and what the plan was for her upon discharge from that facility. Mara answered all of Terri's questions. Some facilities require the case management department to conduct the initial assessment within twenty-four hours of admission, but apparently that facility's requirements were different. Prior to her hospitalization, Denise was independent with activities of daily living and would prefer to return to her house, or her second choice was to go to Mara's house when she was stable for discharge.

Mara continued to follow up with the nurses and physicians about her mother's status. She called daily for labs, vital signs, progress with the ventilator, progress with the coma program and her mother's general status. Denise's vital signs fluctuated.

***

March 8, 2017

From day to day, the amount of information that Mara was provided, depended on the person who was giving the information. She appreciated the time that they took to provide the information. One day, about fifteen minutes after she entered the facility, her mother's nurse, Dana, slowly entered the room. She updated Mara on Denise's status. Denise's white blood cell count was elevated and the sputum and blood culture results indicated that she had infections in the blood as well as in the lungs. The physician consulted the infectious disease physician. Contact isolation continued. The staff and visitors were to wear disposable gowns to help prevent the spread of the infection to themselves and to other patients.

The old gastrostomy or feeding tube site in Denise's abdomen was leaking. Medications were seeping out of the opening in her abdomen. A collection bag was placed at the site by the physician and the output was being measured by the nurses. The gastroenterologist was consulted, and he decided that the medications should be administered through the jejunostomy part of the gastrostomy-jejunostomy (GJ) tube. This type of tube has two ports, the gastrostomy (G) port which accesses the stomach and the jejunostomy (J) port accesses the small intestine.

Initially, one of the nurses told Mara that the physician ordered that the medications via the g-tube be minimized, but as the output increased, the physician's order changed to reflect that nothing should be administered via that tube, and everything should be administered via the j-tube. Even though issues with the feeding tube were reoccurring, the nurses did not seem to be concerned enough to be more cautious with it. Mara thought that some of the problems with the feeding tube could have been avoided. Flushing the tube before and after medication administration was important. The medications that required being crushed by the nurses before they were flushed in the tube, needed to be crushed into tiny particles to prevent the tube from being clogged. Again, Mara resorted to thinking things through with her inner voice … *if the same behavior is being performed repeatedly and the same negative outcome is observed, shouldn't logical reasoning suggest a change in behavior?* Was it starting all over again?

Similarly, when Denise was repositioned in the bed while she was connected to various tubes and lines, staff would be expected to be mindful of dislodging any of those tubes. *She should be getting better care,* Mara thought. *I want to see her recover. What is going on? Is this how care is in most places?* This, she thought, is frightening.

Chapter 17

To care or not to care

As she continued to visit her mother every day, Mara noticed that her mother had a significant amount of thick mucus as the nurses and respiratory therapists suctioned her. Denise was getting stronger but was not strong enough to expectorate the mucus. Mara had asked the intensivist to order chest physiotherapy (chest PT) to help break up the mucus and to clear her mother's lungs. The attending physician ordered chest PT to be administered by respiratory therapy. Mara quietly wondered, *so I must try to figure things out with the help of my aunts and then convey the suggestions to the facility*. Certain things were just not included in the plan of care. They operated on a different timeline than Mara thought that they would. She was usually not present at the bedside when the respiratory therapist administered chest physiotherapy.

On one evening, she was there when it all happened. Denise was asleep. As Mara sat at her mother's side, a light-complexioned African

American woman, in her mid-forties, approximately 5ft 7in tall, with short curly black hair, strolled into the room. She had a serious expression on her face. She did not make eye contact with Mara. She placed her clipboard on the computer in the room. She donned the isolation gown that she had taken from the rack on the door and walked over to the ventilator, still not saying a word. She dealt with the ventilator. At that point, Mara assumed that she was the respiratory therapist based on the amount of attention that she paid to the ventilator. She then proceeded to the bed. As she approached the bed, she looked at Mara but did not acknowledge her, until she walked over to the other side of the bed where Mara sat.

"Excuse me, I need to turn this on," the therapist said coldly.

The therapist changed the setting on the bed to chest physiotherapy and immediately the bed started to vibrate. Denise woke up immediately. She quickly reached for the side rail with her right hand. She opened her eyes wide and appeared to Mara to be frightened. Mara sat for a moment with her mouth opened. She made an involuntary movement forward. In her nursing training, she had been taught to identify herself to her patients and to inform them about the care that she would provide to them. Mara thought that she only noticed this repeated behavior from one facility to another because she was present at the bedside when it occurred.

"It's okay Mummy," Mara said gently, as she leaned forward quickly comforting her mother. "You're okay. Just try to relax okay, the bed is vibrating because you're having chest PT, this is one step closer to getting off the vent."

Mara glanced at the therapist and decided to introduce herself since it appeared she wouldn't say anything at all.

"Hi I am Mara. I'm Denise's daughter."

"Yes, I've seen you before," she replied, still stoic and without warmth. "I'm…"

Mara did not catch the name. She looked to see if the therapist were wearing a badge but realized that it was turned around so Mara could not see the name. The respiratory therapist's attention was entirely focused on the computer in the room. Mara hesitated.

"Can you tell me… the duration for the chest PT?" she asked.

"About ten minutes…" the therapist replied, without taking even a brief moment to turn her attention from the computer screen.

Mara looked at her mother in the bed. Her eyes were still wide open—still shocked by the shaking bed that woke her. She rubbed her mother's arm. *So, this is why they say she has anxiety. Wouldn't this therapist be frightened if she were asleep in the bed, and it started to vibrate? I really don't want to create any problems for mummy, but I need to say something to this lady, —especially if she's going to work with her again.* Is a person who cannot use their voice a non-person? Is this how we do caregiving everywhere? Why haven't I noticed this before Mummy became ill? Mara cleared her throat and looked over at the therapist, who was still typing on the computer keyboard.

"You know, in order for my mom to have less anxiety, I would like for her to be informed before any care is administered."

The therapist paused, kept her eye on the computer screen, as she widened her lips to the sides in an obvious performance of a non-smile. She only said, "okay."

The speed of the vibration on Denise's bed slowed down. The therapist closed the computer screen, walked over to the side of the bed, and pressed a button. The vibrations stopped completely. She picked up her clipboard from the computer and walked towards the door, removed her isolation gown, placed it in the trash can and walked out of the room.

Mara was trying to process what just happened. *You do not question power, I guess, whatever level it comes from. You do not question authority.*

Mara wanted to make sure that the type of care that she had seen her mother receive from the therapist did not continue. She walked out of the room and went to the pod table where her mother's nurse and three others were sitting.

"Can I speak with the charge nurse?" she asked.

The nurse assigned to Denise stood up, "Sure. Is there something with which I can help?"

"Well, I actually need to speak with both of you," Mara sighed.

The nurse called the charge nurse on the phone, "Hey Betty, can you come over here? I am with Ms. Mitchell's daughter, and she wants to speak with you."

The nurse hung up the receiver and Mara stood in front of the pod table for a few minutes when Betty, the charge nurse, walking briskly down the hallway approached them. Betty extended her hand and introduced herself, "Hi, I am Betty. I'm in charge this evening."

Mara shook Betty's hand. "I am Mara. Ms. Mitchell's daughter. My mom was asleep, and the respiratory therapist just started chest PT without saying anything to her to let her know what to expect. I would like my mother to be informed prior to care being provided."

"I'm sorry," Betty responded. "I will talk to the nursing staff and pass it on in report. Okay? I am sorry."

Mara, feeling frustrated that she had to constantly advocate, said to Betty, "thank you" and walked back into her mother's room. She knew that she could not be always at her mother's side but when certain factors were obviously contributing to the nurses medicating her mother for anxiety without reason, it was her duty, she felt, to say something. She saw no point in allowing staff to create additional problems for the sake of medicating her mother.

Mara told herself that she needed to be careful because she could not be there every second. This surely was a problem for other patients and not only her mother. Were pharmaceutical companies profiting from all this improper care? Of course, she was anxious and she needed proper care, not to be medicated for anxiety.

***

Denise was now experiencing quite a few complications. Neurologically, she was slow to respond, but she was a fighter and she made significant efforts to respond appropriately. Respiratory related, she was making progress with the ventilator but had started the entire process all over once she transferred to that facility. The doctors treated her for pneumonia at least twice. She continued to have edema. She remained in acute renal failure and dialysis continued. Mara was pleased, though, to see the improvements that her mother had made, especially with her kidney function. She considered the trend in the kidney function tests and appreciated the results every time the physicians ordered laboratory tests. Denise had not been able to produce urine for a while and had now started doing so again. She was able to move all her extremities except her left arm and hand. Her left hand was not only affected by the stroke and unable to move but the fingers were curled inward and painful if anyone attempted to exercise them. There was a splint that the staff should have applied daily based on the occupational therapists' recommendation at Northern Metropolitan Hospital, but it went unnoticed by the nurses and therapists at the Baltimore facility. There was no physician's order to address the left hand, so it was completely ignored by the staff.

Mara felt like she was being a constant bother, but if she ignored the issue then her mother's hand would remain with a contracture. She spoke with the occupational therapist who worked with her mother in the coma program. The therapist assured her that she would speak with the nurses and would also post at the bedside a schedule for the application of the splint.

Chapter 18

Itching versus anxiety

On the evening of the same day that Mara spoke with the occupational therapist about her mother's splint, Mara noticed that the schedule for the splint was posted above the head of her mother's bed. Based on the schedule, the splint was—and should be off.

The next day, Mara was off from her job. She visited her mother earlier in the day and observed that the staff provided care as expected. The staff responded in a timely manner to the call bell whenever Mara called for assistance. She called for issues such as when the tube feeding bag needed to be changed, the intravenous antibiotic bag was completed and when her mother needed to be suctioned. Her mother's arms were elevated on the pillows. The next few days were about the same. Care was appropriate. For several consecutive days, her mother's daytime nurse was Dana. The nurses worked overtime frequently. Mara was concerned about the nurses being exhausted and unable to perform as they should while her mother was under their care. Of course, she was concerned not only about her mother. As she realized how often each nurse was scheduled, she wondered whether they were getting enough rest. There were no nursing issues while Dana remained the nurse who was assigned to her mother.

***

On April 10, 2017, Dialysis continued. The kidney function tests continued to improve. Mara called the unit and spoke with her mother's nurse, Darielle. The multidisciplinary team did not meet to discuss the care of every patient daily, also known as rounds in the hospital setting. The team rounded on each patient on scheduled days. It was Monday. This was the day that the team rounded on Denise. The plan was for the intensivist to follow up with the nephrologist as there was a possibility that dialysis would be skipped that day. Mara was certainly hopeful that her mother would no longer need to have dialysis. She was pleased to see the improvements her mother had made. The possibility that her renal function was almost at baseline was an answer to many prayers. Mara spoke with Darielle later in the evening when she arrived at the facility.

Darielle had a very stoic expression and Mara thought her tone was quite harsh as she provided updates about the events of her mother's day. Had something happened? After completing a terribly busy day at work and having a long drive to visit her mother, Mara tried not to internalize the unpleasant attitudes that she was beginning to sense from some members of the staff. Were there issues related to the care of her mother? They were at work, too—so were there other issues? Mara tried to remain professional and to merely show concern about her mother's status. Perhaps the staff was not familiar with families who were interested in being involved, who showed that they cared about a loved one, and, importantly, who knew enough to ask pertinent questions. She was beginning to get that feeling here, too—that she was asking too many questions. Was this normal? Was something wrong with her approach? She thought of how they responded to family queries at her institution. Was this conflict between family and facility inevitable? Would those who asked few questions always be the "good" patients? But didn't nurses who worked also have families? Have they ever been frightened, worried, and frustrated as they watched a loved one struggle to stay alive? Or perhaps they had not, yet?

Darielle told Mara that the nephrologist decided that dialysis was not necessary that day, but she did not seem happy to deliver news that was positive, that her patient's daughter would be happy to receive. A few more days passed. Based on the laboratory tests for kidney function, dialysis was skipped again. The dialysis catheter remained in place in Denise's right upper chest, if it would be needed.

On April 17, 2017, Denise began to experience itching, mostly near the dialysis catheter site. Her nurse Pamela told Mara that she and other nurses on the unit were concerned that Denise would inadvertently pull out the dialysis catheter as she tried to relieve the itching by scratching the area. The nurses applied a mitten to the right hand to prevent her from pulling out the catheter. That was also their solution to the itching. At some facilities, nurses need a doctor's order before placing mittens on patients. Was there a doctor's order for the mittens? If a doctor's order were required, Mara thought that the doctor would be informed or would be interested to know the purpose of the mitten. If the doctor was made aware of the itching, might he or she not order something to relieve the itching? Nothing made sense, but Mara tried to make sense of it all. She continued to visit her mother every day after work.

The first day that her mother showed signs of discomfort with itching, Mara noticed the mitten. She inquired from the nurse and the explanation was that her mother could hurt herself if she pulled out the catheter. Mara agreed that if the catheter were pulled out it could cause trauma to her mother. She found it disturbing that the nurse did not see the need to obtain an order for an antihistamine such as Benadryl to help relieve the itching. Should she ask? Her mother seemed more uncomfortable the longer she was forced to deal with the itching. She started to hit the siderail with her right hand. She was medicated for anxiety with Seroquel. Why did these facilities seem so quick to give medication for anxiety? Couldn't they try to stop the itching? Might you not hit against the bedrail if you were trying not to scratch? She could not understand why certain things were occurring. Would it have been easier or better if she were not visiting her mother and was unaware of the care that was being provided? For whom would it have been easier or better? Denise was unable to move her left hand due to the strokes. Her dominant hand was the right. She was on the ventilator and unable to speak. She was, however, able to mouth some of her words. She needed help to be relieved from the annoying discomfort of itching and there was no one in the room apart from her roommate who was also on the ventilator. To get attention and to relieve the frustration and discomfort, she found it necessary to hit the side of the rail of her bed. Her behavior did not seem unreasonable to Mara, but was it a problem for the nurses? Mara tried to process the logic behind all the things that were occurring. It was an impossible task. Why medicate her for anxiety? There was a clear difference between itching and anxiety. Finally, she informed the nurse that she would like her to obtain an order for Benadryl. Perhaps the nurses did not believe that Denise was experiencing itching? Or was it just a lack of imagination? Wasn't it that they would do at home? Try to relieve the itching? Did they just not care? At least they could try something. It might work. An order was given by the attending physician for Benadryl to be administered by the nurses.

On April 18, 2017, the following day, Denise continued to exhibit signs of discomfort with itching that was localized to her right upper chest. It was like déjà vu. This time it was a different nurse, Kerry. Denise had once again been medicated by the nurse for anxiety. Nothing was administered for itching. Ordinarily, if a person had the ability to care for self and had itching, the first instinct would be to find something to give relief. Someone under the care of health personnel would have the same expectation but would need to rely on the health care professionals to assist. Again, Mara addressed the issue with her mother's nurse and insisted that her mother's discomfort be relieved. She inquired from her about the Benadryl and was told that it was a one-time order. If there was a specific reason Benadryl was ordered to be administered only once, Mara was open to being educated about it. She was aware that sometimes the providers do not have the time to explain every decision that they make, but if there was a reason, she was interested in knowing what it was, so that it did not remain an unanswered question in her mind. She would ask for an alternative to be considered, for her mother to be comfortable. She could not read minds, she thought in frustration, and so the only way to get answers was to ask questions. She spoke with the attending physician at the bedside, and he ordered Benadryl for her mother, as needed.

On April 19, 2017, the itches continued to be an issue and the nurse administered Benadryl. In the meantime, Denise was still being medicated for anxiety. The staff reported to Mara, as well as to each other, that Denise wanted someone to be always in the room with her and they were not staffed sufficiently to accommodate. As she listened to Kerry the evening nurse's comments, Mara silently thought, *no need to argue, my mother is still under their care.*

At all times? There was absolutely no need for someone to be always in Denise's room. Someone needed to be present in the room long enough to address her immediate needs whatever they were, and it appeared that the most immediate was the itching. Her mother was very sociable, yes. She enjoyed the company of others, but she was also able to decipher uncaring, unprofessional, and indignant attitudes. Mara was sure she would not want unpleasant people in her room. Mara informed Kerry that she would remove the mitten while she visited; Kerry approved.

April 20, 2017, the next day, Mara was told by her mother's nurse that the doctor discontinued the Benadryl, because it made her mother 'sleep too much'. Of course, thought Mara. The nurses were medicating her with both Benadryl and Seroquel. One would expect her to be drowsy. Give her the Benadryl and discontinue the anxiety medication! Angry now, Mara reflected that one did not need a college degree to figure that out. If a combination of two medications that can cause drowsiness was administered to someone, who was medically compromised, drowsiness was guaranteed. On the other hand, the drowsiness may have solved the staff's concern about their patient wanting someone to be always in her room. It was difficult to determine what the staff wanted.

So, she needed to do something. On the following evening, Mara brought a few topical anti-itching creams, Benadryl, calamine, and Aveeno to her mother's room. She informed the nurse that she would apply one of them to her mother's skin. The nurse granted permission. She started with the Benadryl lotion and applied it to her mother's right upper chest near the dressing of the dialysis catheter. The night nurse came on duty and was concerned that the lotion would cause the dressing to peel off. It was a pity that the nurse's and Mara's concerns differed. Mara informed Kimberly, the nurse, that perhaps there was another type of dressing that could be used to replace the current one. She inquired about whether the nurses or physicians discussed what they thought could be causing her mother to itch. Kimberly informed her that she only worked the night shift and asked whether Mara had spoken to someone on the day shift about that issue. As Mara recalled, prior to her mother's transfer to the Baltimore long term acute care hospital, Maribeth informed her that a physician would be always on duty. If that information were true, that meant that Kimberly had access to a physician or a physician assistant during her shift. Kimberly's response suggested that Mara was responsible for getting direct answers to her questions from the providers, that she should not rely on her assistance to get those answers. The conversation, Mara thought, was a very strange one. Mara suggested that her mother was reacting to the tape or to the dressing that covered the dialysis catheter. Kimberly was frustrated. Her attitude suggested that Mara should figure out such things herself. She suggested that Mara call the following morning to speak with someone on the day shift.

Okay. So, you do not see this as your job, and this is not your mother. She is my mother. She planned to take Kimberly's advice. Mara spent a little more time visiting her mother. She applied some more lotion to her mother's skin, performed some exercises with her, lifting her arms and then each foot and said a prayer. Someone announced on the intercom system that visiting hours had ended. She kissed and hugged her mother goodnight and headed for home. On her way out of the building, she saw the security guard whom she had not seen since the first night, at the front desk. He was very pleasant and wished her a good night. She was not violating visiting hours. Mara sent out text messages as she did every night to update family and friends and to request prayers for her mother.

The next morning, Mara called the unit where her mother was located and requested to speak with the physician. She was placed on hold by someone whom she clearly had interrupted. The facility's human resources department contributed to society by providing jobs for individuals in the community; however, their contribution was incomplete. Mara thought that they needed to ensure that their employees had proper phone etiquette, especially in that setting. Her mother's nurse, Dana, came on the phone. Dana updated Mara about her mother's progress. Dana said that she had applied Aveeno to Denise's chest and it seemed to have helped. She told Mara that she asked the nursing assistants to apply the Aveeno after Denise's morning care; they had, and Denise was asleep at that moment. Mara thanked Dana. She expressed to Dana that she thought that the dressing that covered the dialysis catheter or the tape was causing the itching. Dana told her that it was possible and that she would convey her concern to the physician who was not on the unit at that moment. Mara also learned from a colleague that sometimes patients who were on dialysis experience itching but an actual cause was not provided. It was not satisfactory to know that patients on dialysis experienced itching. There must be an actual cause and a solution. Later that afternoon, Mara received a phone call from the attending physician who said that he had spoken with the nephrologist, and they decided that Denise would not continue with dialysis. Her kidney was continuing to recover, and the staff would remove the dialysis catheter.

Chapter 19

End of dialysis

As she processed the news about the end of dialysis, Mara could not help but recall her conversation with Dr. Kennedy at the Northern Metropolitan Hospital. Her mother, who was in multiorgan failure and should have been placed on hospice per Dr. Kennedy's suggestion, had been placed on dialysis instead and her kidney function was recovering. This was approximately three months later. If it had been one of his family members whose life he *valued* or another patient whom he thought was *worth* the effort of his medical care, would his suggestion have been the same?

Mara visited her mother after work that evening. Denise was in good spirits. She seemed comfortable. She moved her extremities to show her daughter how much she was able to do independently. Dana entered the room and provided Mara with Denise's vital signs and laboratory results. She told Mara that Denise was transferred from the bed to the chair earlier in the day and sat up for a longer period than she had done in the past. Denise heard the entire conversation and seemed proud of herself, as she smiled when she heard the news that was being relayed to her daughter. Dana had a serious expression most times when she met Mara, but she provided diligent care to Denise and seemed confident in her role as a nurse. Although she rarely smiled when she saw Mara, there was always a pleasant expression when she spoke to Denise. It was also obvious that Denise liked Dana and was comfortable with her. Mara asked Dana questions and gave her opinions about her mother's status and there was never a frown nor an argument from Dana. Good, thought Mara. *You do not have to like me. Be good to my mother! That works.*

She just wanted Dana to feel as though they were working toward a common goal. Although Dana worked several consecutive days, Mara secretly wished that Dana could be her mother's nurse daily for the duration of her mother's stay at the facility. That was merely dreaming. She wanted her mother and all the other patients to be safe under the care of the health care personnel. It was important that Dana took care of herself and rested well to provide safe care.

The next morning, instead of calling the facility, Mara went to visit her mother earlier in the day as she was off from her job. She met the intensivist, Dr. Nabin, whom she had not met before but with whom she had spoken on the telephone. Dr. Nabin appeared to be a young lady, in her forties, and of South Asian descent. She walked very briskly and her speech, very rapid, seemed made to match. She updated Mara about Denise's status. She discussed the lab results with Mara.

"There is a lot going on with your mother. Her white blood cell count is high. Her hemoglobin and hematocrit are a bit low, and she will need at least one unit of blood. The kidney functions tests, both BUN and creatinine are trending down in the right direction."

The physician paused for a moment and continued to explain, "Her kidneys are recovering, but we're also giving her Lasix to remove excess fluid."

Mara was pleased that despite the excess fluid, her mother did not need dialysis. Dr. Nabin continued, "Her lungs need to rest and so we won't attempt any weaning during this time with all that is happening with her." Whatever was best for her mother was what Mara wanted.

Mara continued to take note of her mother's lab results and reported them to her aunts Ali and Simone, healthcare professionals themselves, who would understand and could advise. The white blood cell count was decreasing.

Denise was on an antibiotic. The kidney function tests continued to improve, and the hemoglobin and hematocrit improved slightly.

As more progress was made with Denise's health, Mara and Denise's visitors noticed the changes. She was clearly improving, although she struggled in some areas. Elevated blood pressure was an issue. More fluid was still being removed. Denise was tolerating the tube feeding without any issues and that was good news as she had many issues with the tube feeding.

Chapter 20

Vent weaning

Mara spoke with the intensivist Dr. Nabin, who notified Mara, "There would not be any more attempts at the weaning trials from the ventilator for your mom at this facility. She can transfer to a nursing home where they can take care of her on the vent."

That was unexpected news. "I'm sorry but I don't understand why that would be," Mara said to Dr. Nabin. "That is why she is here. I thought that the weaning was suspended because she is sick, but you are saying she will not have any more trials. Can you tell me why?"

In Mara's mind, her mother had transferred to that facility specifically to be weaned from the ventilator, so what the physician told her did not make any sense. Mara felt as though she was being a bother by asking for an explanation. "I'll ask the pulmonologist to speak with you," Dr. Nabin said.

Perhaps Dr. Nabin really did not know why the weaning trials would not continue. It was obvious that she wanted the discussion to end even before it had started. The conversation ended with the physician informing Mara, "Let me know if you have any other questions or concerns."

Her mannerisms appeared to suggest that she had no intention of entertaining any more questions or concerns from Mara. There was not much time left for Mara to continue the visit with her mother. She played some music on her cell phone for her mother, who was incredibly happy to hear familiar sounds. The announcement was made on the intercom that visiting hours had ended. She decided to send the group text messages before she started her drive home. Mara said prayers at her mother's side and left her room. She wished the staff outside of the room a good night and extended the same courtesy to the security guard at the front desk. She walked to her car in the parking lot and felt the tears as they just flooded her eyes and rolled down her cheeks. Really, she was at the stage where she did not know what to do. This felt like an uphill battle not just about her mother's care, but against health facilities which had their own competing interests to consider.

The resistance that Mara felt from the health care providers since the day that her mother experienced the angioedema at the Northern Metropolitan Hospital was overwhelming. Everyone seemed to be putting up a wall. They did not even know why they were behaving like that, just that they had to. It was reasonable, Mara thought, that she should ask questions if she were interested in getting answers. Denise was transferred to the facility to be weaned off the ventilator. They attempted to wean her with no success, they had concluded, and without having a conversation with her daughter, the facility decided that she should spend the rest of her life in a nursing home, on a ventilator. Why had they made that decision? How *could* they make that decision without talking to her? The idea of the nursing home was presented by the intensivist Dr. Nabin, at the long-term acute care hospital. Dr. Nabin did not know why her patient's weaning trials would cease, or simply did not care to share that information with Mara. Her expertise, Mara concluded, was in transferring patients to nursing homes. Was this about a financial consideration for the health service? Mara prepared herself mentally to have a conversation with the pulmonologist. She suspected that it would not be an easy conversation, but she refused to be intimidated by a title. She had the utmost respect for everyone, regardless of position; however, her primary concern was her mother.

***

On the morning of May 13, 2017, Mara was at work and received a call from the pulmonologist, Dr. Bandara.

"I just saw your mother. She had a nice smile and appeared to be comfortable," the physician said.

Mara listened quietly. She realized that was the physician's icebreaker. She did not mention Denise's medical condition or the setting on the ventilator. She focused on what she believed her patient's daughter would be pleased to hear. Mara thought, "I know my mother has a nice smile..." and Dr. Bandara did not need to remind her of that. She just wanted to discuss her mother's medical condition and the plans to move forward. There was a moment of silence. "I've decided not to continue with the weaning trials with your mother," Dr. Bandara said. "You know, not every patient gets off the ventilator. Being on the ventilator may be her new baseline. We should not push her because she has been through so much and her lungs need to rest."

Mara continued to listen and resisted the growing urge to interject before she finished. "Also, the insurance would not continue to cover her stay at this facility, as she has been here for a couple of months. We tried to wean her several times without any success."

Such rhetoric, Mara thought made no sense. But this is the issue. Care is about money, and the insurance would not continue to pay beyond a certain time. When the insurance limit is up, so is your time to exist. She prepared to do battle. This was a long-term acute care hospital. Denise transferred to that facility because she required more time to recover. The comment that Dr. Bandara had made regarding insurance coverage may have been an assumption.

Thinking it all through, Mara allowed Dr. Bandara to continue with her story without interruption. As if it was meant to be a monologue, Dr. Bandara said, "Okay. Well, it was nice talking to you. We will continue to take care of your mother."

Some providers have no interest in addressing questions or comments from those whom they provide care to or their families. Mara said to Dr. Bandara, "Actually, I'd like to say something." The physician responded, "Go ahead." Mara forgot to say, 'without interruption.' She told the physician, "I'm not aware of the several times of weaning trials that you referenced." Dr. Bandara was prepared for this conversation as she had dates available with her and presented those dates. Mara also had dates with her and spoke about those dates as they correlated with her mother having infections, pseudomonas at least twice and fluid overload.

Prior to receiving the phone call from the physician, Mara contacted her mother's health insurance company and contacted the nurse case manager, Toni, who was managing her mother's case. It was not an easy task to locate Toni. She made the first call to Denise's employer with a request to be pointed in the right direction. Mara found the staff at her mother's job to be extremely helpful and received a few responses aimed at ensuring that she received the information that she needed. Nurse case manager Toni, explained to Mara that her mother met criteria to continue to receive care at the long-term acute care facility and that she would continue to authorize her stay at the facility.

Now, Mara was able to inform Dr. Bandara. "My mother's stay at the long-term acute care hospital continues to be authorized and she continues to meet criteria to be there," Mara said confidently. "I was told by the insurance company."

It was a phone conversation, so it was not possible to see Dr. Bandara's expression, but from the tone of her voice, she was clearly not happy.

Perhaps Dr. Bandara perceived Mara's responses as disrespectful just because Mara disagreed with her. Perhaps some families did not ask questions or closely monitored their loved one's care or are intimidated by the mysteries of the health care system. For Mara, the question was simple. How could she, as a daughter, ignore her mother who played a significant role in her life? Could she care about her patients or any other person and not care about her own mother? If she found that she could care about others and not advocate for her mother, then she would have had to do some significant soul-searching. Her mother was a part of her. She felt not doing the best for her would be like self-hatred.

Mara imagined that she was labeled by those with whom she was now coming into contact as a difficult daughter. Everything that she did as they pertained to her mother's care came naturally. She could not imagine behaving any differently. She kept thinking that if she did not fight for her mother, who would she be able to depend on to have those difficult conversations. Her mother's friends were incredibly supportive, but they would not be permitted by the facilities to speak on Denise's behalf. The facilities would be concerned about the Health Insurance Portability and Accountability Act (HIPAA). As part of the HIPAA rule, patients' medical records and other personal health information are to be kept confidential. This information could only be shared with Mara as she was her mother's primary agent to speak on her behalf. Mara would not want them to violate this

Act, and neither would her mother. She knew that she could only be professional and polite, as it was her mother's life that was affected. Conducting herself any other way would only be harmful to her mother.

Dr. Bandara stated, very matter-of-factly, "We have tried to wean her." It sounded as though she had done Denise a favor or favors. She told Mara that about five attempts were made to wean her mother. Mara was pleased to hear those attempts had been made; however, she was not expecting those attempts to count against her mother, given the fact that she was not medically stable to be successful at weaning trials. Mara thought that if those attempts were treated as though her mother was given preliminary trials, she would have understood. Her mother's lungs would have been prepared for the real weaning trial when she was stable.

"Well on those occasions when weaning trials were attempted, she had pseudomonas and fluid overload," Mara said, reminding the doctor of what should have been obvious.

In that moment, Mara realized that the conversation had gotten to a point where they both were repeating themselves. It turned into a debate in which neither one was able to convince the other of their points. Mara's arguments were focused on the infections and fluid overload that her mother struggled with. She had dates. She knew when things had happened. Dr. Bandara's arguments were more focused on the number of times that attempts were made at weaning, not on the medical stability of her patient. Normally, Mara thought, the expectation would be that the physician would be concerned about medical stability, preventing complications, and avoiding readmissions. Mara strongly believed that those were certainly not appropriate times for her mother to be weaned, especially if she would not be given other opportunities. Denise was not her strongest self. Unless the expectation was to have her fail, what would be the reason to rush to wean rather than to wait until she was stable? This hospital's designation was "long term acute care" and the insurance was still willing to continue to cover the stay at the facility. So, what was the problem?

***

Mara considered the statistics that Maribeth had provided to her prior to her mother's transfer. The facility expected patients be at a certain level in their recovery process after a pre-calculated amount of time had passed. After a particular period, they were 'not weanable' and that was the description that was now being affixed to Denise. They did not consider the fact that every patient was different and that their bodies responded differently. The fact that Denise had been through so much, as Dr. Bandara informed Mara, was only used to the facility's advantage. It did not occur to the pulmonologist that the point that she made, was the actual reason Denise needed more time to be weaned from the ventilator. It was disappointing to Mara that the facility was merely concerned about maintaining or improving statistics, rather than providing individualized care. Apart from the fact that Denise was a patient at the facility, there was not much else that Mara and Dr. Bandara seemed to agree on. The phone call ended with no promises or expectations on either side. Mara felt that she was not asking for favors or anything impossible. She simply wanted her mother to have a fair chance at weaning from the ventilator. She knew that it was important to have that conversation with Dr. Bandara because she needed to know and understand the physician's rationale. If she had not had the conversation, she would have had regrets and she would always be speculating about what could have been.

Chapter 21

Addressing the issues

On May 13, 2017, as part of her daily routine, Mara placed a call to speak with her mother's nurse. Denise had vomited that morning and was medicated by nurse. An abdominal x-ray was done, and it was discovered that the feeding tube was dislodged. The tube was pulled out of place from her being repositioned in the bed. The dislodged tube explained the pain of which she was complaining. Everything was in slow motion. The cause of the abdominal pain should have been identified sooner; Mara felt. An intensive care facility should be more quickly able to identify these things, and workers should be curious enough to investigate thoroughly. Mara wondered how much more her mother was expected to endure. She had to continuously try to figure things out, whether it was on her own or with the input of her aunts Ali, Simone, or Breana, and then convey their opinions to the facility. If she had not been that involved, what would her mother's care be like? The tube feeding was stopped by the nurses per the doctor's order and there was plan for a new feeding tube. Was there, she wondered, any feeling of unease or responsibility on the part of the facility and its workers?

A chest x-ray was done. Denise had pneumonia. She started on intravenous antibiotics again to treat the pneumonia. A new gastrostomy feeding tube was placed, and the tube feeding was started. The laboratory results were improving. As Mara thought about it all, she realized she was getting into the habit of thinking things through like the health system. It was all about what was being done to or for the patient. A tube *was placed...* A feeding tube *was stopped.* The individual to whom things were being done was hardly visible in all of this. There was a lot happening, but Denise was a fighter, so she fought. She clearly wanted to live. Now that the tube feeding had started, Mara learned from the nurse that her mother was having loose stools. Denise was out of the bed but was only able to tolerate approximately two hours sitting in the chair. She was medicated for the loose stools and the tube feeding rate was decreased. Despite the improvement in her renal function and other labs, the intensivist placed a nephrology consult. She urinated; however, her body was still holding on to excess fluid. The nephrologist suggested that she should be diuresed with Lasix—that is, she should be given Lasix to remove excess fluid. The diuresis was taking effect.

Mara spoke with the intensivist who came on duty for the week, Dr. Bean. The physician stated that she would like to eliminate excess fluids completely and then try to wean Denise from the ventilator again during that week. Mara was pleased to hear that. The loose stools had decreased. Labs were improving. Denise did not have any health-related complaints, other than back pains that she had been complaining about for some time. Mara spoke with her mother and encouraged her to sit in the chair whenever the staff tried to get her up. She hoped that if Denise sat up, the back pain would be less or she would not have them at all. She also hoped that it would help to prevent another onset of pneumonia and that it would help her mother to become stronger and more alert.

Mara was thinking now that there was no consistency in the care that the staff provided to Denise. So much seemed dependent on who was on duty—which intensivist, which pulmonologist, which respiratory therapist and nurse. Although no one at the Baltimore facility would attest to the fact that Denise was not stable for discharge when the discussion had been brought up earlier on by Dr. Bandara and Dr. Nabin, it was clear that she was not ready for discharge at that time. After that initial discussion, there were so many different issues that needed to be addressed. Denise had edema and needed to have excess fluid removed. She had pneumonia and was placed on antibiotics. The gastrostomy tube was dislodged, and she needed to have a new gastrostomy tube placed. She had diarrhea that needed to be resolved. If Denise had left the Baltimore facility at the time when Dr. Bandara was adamant that she would not have any more weaning and when Dr. Nabin suggested that she was to transfer to a nursing home to live, more than likely Denise would have been readmitted at another hospital to address the issues that she was having and that could have been addressed at the long term acute care hospital. The Baltimore facility may not have been interested in Denise, but it had an interest in the thought of avoiding readmission, whether it was there or somewhere else. Concerned for her mother and concerned about the level of care at the facility, Mara took a note to bring that issue up to administration. She realized that while the individuals who were directly involved in her mother's care would have certain areas of focus, administration would look at a broader picture and hopefully make prudent decisions. She had no problem asking for her mother to be readmitted to a hospital if she was not stable in a subacute rehabilitation or skilled nursing facility. She could not help feeling that the fact that the physicians were providing care to an acutely ill patient and were considering having her transfer to a lower level of care, suggested that they truly did not care about that patient. They simply wanted her off their premises. As Mara tried to process it all, she could only believe that they had given up on any possibility of recovery for Denise. She had been down that path before. But she had not given up on her mother's recovery. She could not understand why they would give up. It seemed to her that the Baltimore facility's plan was to transfer her out to another facility, one that would not be able to provide the care that she needed. Again, she wondered—was this about money, about what they thought the insurance would cover? Or were they tired of the things they had to do? Or was it that she, Mara, was asking too many questions and expressing her concerns too frequently?

Mara tried her best to keep all the negative information away from her mother. She avoided having difficult conversations with caregivers in her mother's presence. Her mother needed positive reinforcement. Mara also asked the visitors to do the same. She had no control over what occurred in her absence, but she tried as much as she could to protect her mother.

Chapter 22

Social Worker

Mara was sitting at her desk at work. She received a phone call from the social worker Fecelia, at the Baltimore facility. The call started with Fecelia being very friendly. She said to Mara, "I hope your day is going well. I called to discuss plans for your mom. More like an update. So, since your mom cannot be weaned from the ventilator, it would be best for her to be at a nursing home where she would be cared for."

Mara listened. Fecelia, it seemed, was on a mission. She knew that Fecelia would not be acting on her own. She would be calling on behalf of the hospital and acting in accordance with orders from the physicians Dr. Bandara and Dr. Nabin who were on duty again. Social workers, she knew, would be expected to follow the physicians' orders to start discharge planning. She also knew that ultimately it was the family's decision whether Denise would transfer to a nursing home to live or for short-term rehabilitation.

Mara did not appreciate the fact that the social worker or the physicians were making decisions for her. She thought angrily that neither she nor her mother had relinquished their rights to the facility. The recommendation that Denise should be at a nursing home because, as they claimed, she could not be weaned from the ventilator was an opinion that they were entitled to, but they could not make decisions without consultation with the family. And Mara thought, I do not agree with their assessment. She listened.

Fecelia continued, "I found a facility that is interested in accepting your mother as early as today." Mara stared at the phone. She did not trust herself to speak. She was silent, trying to find what might be the proper tone. Fecelia continued, "I would arrange the transportation to get her to the nursing home. It is called MNT Nursing Home."

Mara thought, *I know about discharge planning. This is not how discharge planning should work. Why is she telling me these things? They have not asked me anything. I have not agreed to have my mother live at a nursing home.*

If her mother must transfer to another facility for short term, would the family have any part in the selection of the facility? Would there be an opportunity for the family to research, visit facilities, speak to others who may know something about these facilities or even consider distance as a factor? Is that the process for this facility to allow the discharge planner to select for the family? Her mother had medical issues that still needed to be addressed. She had improved a lot but was not at the stage where she was ready to be transferred to a lower level of care. She still needed medical attention. They would have to monitor her. Do they normally transfer patients who require medical attention and frequent monitoring to facilities that are not pre-pared to provide those services? What would hap-pen if she were transferred to a facility that does not have the capability of monitoring patients closely and she has an emergency?

"We can go ahead and transfer your mom to MNT Nursing Home," Fecelia told Mara.

Mara knew the facility. There had been talk about it. She remembered that the facility was pro-hibited from accepting patients some months prior, until they made corrective measures on deficiencies that were found by the state. Was this how they trea-ted patients? Could someone who had no knowled-ge of this kind of internal information be railroaded into agreeing to have a relative moved to a facility considered suspect even by the health system? Mara was not willing to have her mother become one of the first patients that the facility accepted once they received permission to re-open. Mara knew that she did not owe an explanation to Fecelia or anyone else. Also, she was not given a list of facilities to choose from. In her mind's eye, she could almost see the instruction brochure that advised, "Provide families with the right healthcare." Clearly, Fecelia had been allowed to make choices for families in the past. Or had not families been given an opportunity to participate in the decision-making process? Are families made aware that there are other facilities, and they have choices? The moment that Fecelia seemed as though she needed to take a breath between words, Mara decided that she would take the opportunity to inform her of her plans for her mother.

"The plan is not for my mother to be transferred to a nursing home...." Mara said authoritatively.

Fecelia quickly responded, "I am sorry, I am sorry. I cannot understand you. I cannot understand."

Several thoughts entered Mara's mind: *Why wouldn't she be able to understand me? At times like this, I always wonder if there is some intention. Is it an opportunity to say something about a West Indian accent? Truth is, I am never sure.*

Now Mara felt the way she felt when she heard one of her own co-workers comment that, "West Indians like to come here." What was that type of behavior? Was that xenophobia in the healthcare setting? How does that work in terms of patient care? The Washington, D.C. metropolitan area is a diverse area with multiple languages spoken and various accents. If Fecelia was unable to understand someone who only spoke English—but simply had a different accent from hers, that would be problematic for the discharge planning process.

"I will have to call you back," Fecelia said, abruptly ending the phone call.

Mara tried to understand what just happened. She felt this was yet another demonstration of a healthcare team member performing a monologue when contacting family. Mara saw no point in having a *conversation* with that social worker again.

Mara called the facility's operator and asked to be transferred to the director of the social work department. She had been given the director's number by another social worker, Terri, earlier on but could not seem to find the number in that moment. She was in shock after listening to Fecelia and could not concentrate. It was difficult to do all this while at work. She was unable to call soon after Fecelia's phone call because she was busy at work. The operator transferred her to the director's office. The phone rang a few times and went to voicemail. Mara left a message and requested a return call by Monday morning, as it was already Friday afternoon. While she awaited a response from the director of social services at the facility, Mara decided this was an emergency and she would have to write to administration. This was her mother's life.

Mara's letter to the administration described in detail the distress her mother was in—from the itching, general discomfort, lack of attention, and lack of rehabilitative care. In her opinion, the sub-standard care was a true emergency that impacted her mother's ability to achieve baseline. The baseline being an independent working woman, living on her own. Wasting no time, Mara sent the letter via registered mail.

***

On May 15, 2017, Mara considered that the nursing manager on the unit may not have been aware of the type of care that her mother was receiving. She decided to write an additional letter via email to the nursing manager to provide an update.

Dear Shawna,

I hope that you had an enjoyable weekend and that this email finds you well.

I am sending this email just to keep you informed about issues related to my mother, Denise Mitchell (room 193B). It stems from phone calls that I have received from the social worker Fecelia Stratton regarding plans for discharge. I have left a message for her director (it was already late on Friday when I did so) requesting a phone call and that this social worker no longer contacts me. My mother is having medical issues that need to be addressed. Her JG tube was dislodged over the weekend and replaced with a G tube on Sunday, May 14th. On Friday, May 12th, Fecelia said that my mother would be discharged on Monday, May 15th. I have been trying to explain to Fecelia and to the physicians that my mother continues to have abdominal pain. She also has some edema. In addition, I have learned that the last CXR showed worsening right lung infiltrate. I am attaching a copy of the letter that I have sent to a few members of the management team.

Thanks for your time.

Sincerely,

Mara Mitchell

***

At approximately 9:15am on Monday morning, Mara received a call from Cynthia Blanch, the director of social work at the Baltimore facility. Cynthia was cordial and sounded as though she was eager to hear about the purpose of the call. In the voicemail message, Mara did not provide much information other than a request for a phone call and to have Fecelia reassigned away from her mother's case. She was grateful that the director returned her call, without being provided a more detailed reason in the voicemail. Mara introduced herself as Denise's daughter. She explained to her about her mother's challenges over the last several months and the progress that her mother had made. She stated her plans for her mother and the many roadblocks that they had encountered. She informed her of the conversation that she had with one of her employees, Fecelia. Mara asked the director, "Are you able to understand me?" Cynthia responded, "Yes, I can understand you." Mara told Cynthia that she would like Fecelia to be removed from her mother's case and would like to request that a different social worker who would not have difficulty understanding her be assigned to her mother's case. Cynthia provided two names of social workers, Stacey, and Emily. She told Mara that it would be one of those two ladies who would contact her.

Later that afternoon, Mara received a call from Stacey, who introduced herself as the social worker who was assigned to Denise's case. Stacey asked a few questions, some of the same ones that Terri asked in the initial assessment. Mara thought that Stacey sounded overly excited, but she Mara did not share the excited feeling. Stacey told Mara the call was just for her to introduce herself and that they would discuss plans later. She provided Mara with her phone number but said that she would follow up with the physician to determine when Denise would be ready for discharge and would call after she received more information.

Mara was at her desk at work when she received a call on her personal cell from a number that she did not recognize. She picked up, "hello." On the other end there was a friendly voice, "Hi is this, Mara?" Uncertain if it was a telemarketer, Mara hesitated but then responded, "yes, it is." The other person then said, "this is Melissa from MNT Nursing Home. Your mother has been accepted at MNT Nursing Home." Mara replied, "Thanks but my mom will not be transferred to MNT Nursing Home." The liaison seemingly confused said, "I spoke with the social worker at the Baltimore Long Term Acute Care facility, and she said that your mother is being transferred to MNT. Would you mind telling me why she is not coming to MNT?" By then, Mara thought that the conversation had taken a bizarre turn with her being asked to provide an explanation. She said, "Thanks for accepting my mom. Yes, I do mind. I will only say to you that my mom is not coming to MNT. It looks like I missed a couple of calls from your facility. Please refrain from calling me again. I am sorry but I am at work. I must get back."

Later that day after work, Mara saw her mother, who smiled when her daughter entered the room and did not take her eyes off her. Mara performed some exercises with her mother. Denise indicated when she was too tired to do any more leg lifts by shaking her head 'no.' Mara massaged her mother's upper and lower extremities. Mara called her grandmother's house in Grenada via facetime. Denise smiled when she saw her family and heard their voices. Denise's mother gave her encouraging words and told her that she was praying for her. Her mother, like she always did, told her, "God is love." Denise agreed and started to become sleepy. Her sister, sister-in-law, and brothers all wished her a goodnight. After the call, Mara said prayers at her mother's side as usual and continued to sit there for a bit longer. Denise closed her eyes and dozed off to sleep. Mara left when visiting hours ended.

Chapter 23

Communication

The next day, Mara was at work and Stacey called, "I am working on discharge plans. Remember that MNT Nursing Home is interested in her? We will have to transfer her there because we don't want to lose the bed."

Speaking in a forceful whisper, "My mom is not to be transferred without my permission!" Mara said, as she quickly got up from her desk then marched down the hallway on the unit.

"Interesting choice of words," Stacey responded. "If the physician says that your mother is ready for discharge, then she *would* be transferred to MNT Nursing Home..."

Stacey was prepared for a fight of some kind. But could a social worker do that? Was this usual? She spoke with such authority and certainty. This sounds like a threat, Mara thought. If the transfer is done without permission, can it be considered kidnapping? MNT Nursing Home is aware that the patient's daughter refused the transfer during the phone call with their liaison the previous day.

"Okay, I will be in touch. Bye." Stacey said.

Mara pressed her right hand against her forehead, as tears welled in her eyes. She thought about the entire process. *If mummy is transferred without my permission, I would have a different type of conversation with the facility.*

***

Mara continued to visit her mother daily. Aunt Myrna and another of Denise's friends, Sheryl, suggested that Mara take an occasional break from seeing her mother. In her place, they told her, they would visit. They could see that Mara felt guilty if she missed a day of visiting her mother. Mara was not sure. Still, she knew that she was exhausted. She appreciated the offer.

Mara also thought about her mother. She imagined that it would be good for her mother to have her friends visit her. She reasoned that could even help with her mother's recovery.

Aunt Myrna texted Mara during her visit to update her on the events of Denise's day:

She is very aware. Earlier, when the machine was making sounds, she pointed in that direction, to tell me that is where it was coming from. When I checked and told her the numbers were okay, she nodded.

Aunt Myrna then called Mara on the phone to discuss in more detail about Denise's care—the settings on the ventilator, vital signs and about the speech therapist's session. The blood pressure was elevated. Her mother was transferred by the nursing staff from the bed to the chair via a hoyer lift. After being confined to the bed for several months, Denise became accustomed to being in the bed, and she was unable to tolerate sitting in the chair for prolonged periods of time. Although she was transferred to the chair daily, the duration was short for each occasion. She was afraid of heights; her face said that the whole situation was unusual and frightening, and so once she was placed in the hoyer lift, she panicked, afraid that she would fall. Mara felt sure that this was why her heart rate and blood pressure increased. The nurses had their own form of panic, Mara thought. She felt frustrated that their response was to administer anti-anxiety medications. Didn't they talk to patients? Couldn't they sit and be kind to her, reassure her, let her know they were there and would assure her safety? It would take extra time. Was there no time for intense personal care in these facilities? She thought about work and nurses at her own facility. Was this how things were? Was there something wrong in the system? Was there time to provide individualized care?

Denise was now often drowsy. The speech therapist expressed frustration and lacked the patience to work with a drowsy patient. That frustration was evident in her sessions with Denise. Mara thought...but she *must* be drowsy! They are medicating her.

When Mara visited, she encouraged her mother to 'stay the course.' Mara smiled when her mother very obviously rolled her eyes. Good. At least she was able to do that! There was a time when she could not even open her eyes. Even though her mother had aphasia (and so what visitors would see, she could not put words together) she had improved significantly. Even without words, it was obvious. Denise's many visitors noted the improvements that she had made, and they complimented and encouraged her. Once, when she was in the room, Mara heard her mother's friend, Andrina say, "What! A lot is happening, I declare! You are writing now?" Because indeed Denise sometimes motioned to be given a pad so that she could scribble some idea or question on it. Is the television working? Did you talk to Enid at my job?

The visitors signed the quilt that Auntie Breana made for her. It was a lovely red and black quilt. Denise's progression seemed to Mara to correspond with the number of visitors that she received. There were moments when it was obvious that she was sleepy but wanted to hear the conversations of her visitors, so she tried to force herself to stay awake. Andrina worked at the same organization as Denise. She said to Mara, "I was in the office until 9:30 last night." Denise raised her eyebrow with what Mara interpreted as surprise. Mara responded, "that is late. Why so late?" Andrina continued, "Girl, a lot of work. It is just a busy time."

Denise kept her eyes on Andrina and Mara believed that her mother wanted to participate in the conversation. "That is how it has been for the past several days. It is busy," Andrina continued. "Denise, just get better so you can come back and have some fun in the office, okay. It is time to come back to work."

Denise shook her head from side to side. Mara wondered, *is she frustrated about being here on the bed or is she upset that Andrina has been working late? It is possible it is about Andrina because she worries so much.* The conversation changed when the monitor alarmed and the nurse Sherry came in, looked at Denise and said, "Are you okay Ms. Mitchell?" Denise smiled and nodded to indicate yes. They remained silent for a bit and Denise eventually drifted off to sleep.

Denise was not able to tolerate the passy-muir speaking valve, a device that is attached to the outer opening of the tracheostomy tube and is commonly used to help patients speak more normally. The speaking valve was used when the speech and respiratory therapists worked with her. She experienced coughing spells that lasted for several minutes, whenever they connected the valve to the tracheostomy tube. Mara watched her mother. She could see her struggle when this happened. What must it feel like, not being able to reach people by talking, not being able to explain? They were still using a mitten for her hand. It prevented her from scratching or trying to remove the tube. But what was really going on? Could she talk to her, Mara wondered, to find out what was really going on? Sometimes, when she visited, she removed the mitten and her mother seemed to be more comfortable.

Even though the dialysis catheter was no longer in place, Darielle, the day nurse, was concerned that Denise would scratch at the site and that she was 'banging' on the siderails. There was a discoloration on her right upper chest where the dialysis catheter was removed but the same tape was applied to the area. Mara spoke to the evening nurse Rose.

"I think this tape and or the dressing need to be changed," Mara said, as she continued to apply the Benadryl and aveeno to the area.

Rose was quite pleasant, and happily cleaned the area on Denise's chest, changed the type of dressing and tape and applied some aveeno lotion near the area again. Denise smiled, nodded and while there was no sound, her lips mouthed the words 'thank you.'

Yes! Mara felt a small triumph. She was correct. Her mother needed attention like this. There were trivial things that could be done to make a huge difference.

***

Mara played music for her mother from her cell phone and Denise appeared to enjoy it; she smiled when she recognized the ones she liked. When Mara played Lauren Daigle's "Trust in You," Denise smiled. She began to mouth the words. Mara played a variety of music, and her mother had no objections with the change from one type to another. In no order, she played soca, calypso, gospel, christian music, and rhythm and blues. Mara moved her mother's left arm to the sound of the music and encouraged her.

"Okay Mummy, move your right arm the same way."

Denise lifted her right arm as many as ten times at the sounds of the beat, pointing toward the ceiling. After they were done with the arms, they did the same with the legs. Denise needed support with the left leg. Mara supported her mother's left heel and helped her to move her left leg to the sound of the music ten times. She then said to her mother, "okay, you can do the right." Denise lifted her right leg to the sound of the music as high as she was able to. When it seemed to Mara that her mother was tired, she encouraged her to rest. Denise began to tap with her right hand as she continued to listen to the music. Staff came in periodically to check on her and there were no issues. An intercom voice announced the end of visiting hours. As usual, Mara prayed at her mother's side, wished her a good night, and left. She thanked the staff on her way out, said good night to the lady at the front desk and drove home.

Mara sent out group text messages to update family and friends:

Hello everyone, mummy was in good spirits today. She is alert and responds appropriately. She mouths her words but there is no sound due to the trach. She has had some setbacks that have prevented her from being weaned off the vent at Baltimore Long Term Acute Care facility. While she appears to have made significant progress, she has to transfer to a subacute rehab facility to continue with the weaning process. It has not been decided when and where she will transfer to. Thanks for the continued prayers and support.

***

The following morning, Mara visited her mother earlier in the day. The nurse and nursing assistants were about to attach Denise to the hoyer lift. That was the equipment that resembled or functioned as a crane to transfer patients out of bed, when they were not able to transfer themselves. Mara looked at her mother's face. Her expression said, 'save me.' Mara reassured her, "Mummy you are okay. It's okay. They are just transferring you to the chair. You need to sit up in the chair." Denise did not immediately stop panicking; she was tearful and terrified. One of the nursing assistants suggested, "I think we should either leave her in the bed or give her some medication." Quietly, Mara disagreed, "No I do not think that either one will help her. She needs to sit up in the chair." She continued to speak to her mother, "Mummy you are safe, okay. It is okay."

It took a few minutes, but Denise's rapid breathing slowed down and she allowed the staff to place her in the hoyer lift and transfer her to the chair. Mara sat next to her mother and updated her on stories that she missed. She gave her messages from family and friends who were not able to visit but sent their regards. Denise nodded and smiled in response to the messages. As Denise was adjusting to the tracheostomy tube, Mara learned to read her mother's lips. They kept an entire conversation in which Denise was catching up to events and stories that she had missed.

There was now a little sound from Denise's airway and Mara, when she listened closely, could hear the words her mother spoke. She paid close attention to Denise's lips as Denise asked about specific people such as her friend Josie in Texas and Mara told her that her friend was doing well and sent her regards. She told her that Josie's daughter had traveled from Boston to visit her. Denise asked about her cousin Betty in New York and Mara reminded her that Betty and two of her children were recently there to visit and then she smiled and said, "oh yes."

This was good. She really was improving. She had no trouble with long term memory, but her short-term memory was affected. Denise asked about her friend, Jenice. Now that she was feeling better and more able to communicate, she was asking about everybody. Mara told her that her friend was well. Denise lifted her eyebrows and as if to convey a warning, she told Mara, "but you know, she's afraid of the hospital." They both smiled.

As Denise sat in the chair, Mara encouraged her mother to perform some exercises. She put on some music on her phone and encouraged her mother to move her arms to the music. Mara looked closely and exclaimed, "you're moving your hand!" Denise lifted her left hand about an inch from the arm of the recliner chair that she was sitting in. Mara smiled and quietly thought, *you just need encouragement and you will be okay.*

Chapter 24

Is anyone listening

On May 19, 2017, Mara's and Malcolm's father traveled from Florida to Maryland. From their conversations, Mara realized that he wanted to support them—her and Malcolm and to see Denise, of course, and to use the time to see something of the city. All three visited Denise, who was pleased to see him.

Mara stood next to her mother's bed, and she began to make plans in her mind. She tried to decide how to manage her time while her father visited. She thought to herself, *right now, mummy is my priority. She really needs me. I know that dad will understand that most of my time must be spent with mummy.* They continued to visit until Denise drifted off to sleep. Then they left.

The next morning, prior to going to the Baltimore facility, the three went to visit the museums in Washington, D.C. Mara was not interested in exhibits. *Was it the natural history museum we just came in? I do not even know.* She walked slowly behind her father and brother as they strolled into the gift shop on the lower level of the museum. Her mind was on her mother. *Hopefully, mummy is okay and is not worrying. She is probably wondering if we are coming to visit her today. I am glad that dad is here, but I need to see mummy. We can only visit the museums for a couple of hours and then we must go to see her. She is the one who is sick and needs support, so I have to stay committed.*

About fifteen minutes after they entered the museum's gift shop, Mara's cell phone rang. It was Stacey, the social worker at the long-term acute care hospital.

"Your mother will be transferred to MNT Nursing Home. I obtained authorization from the insurance for transportation."

Mara walked out of the gift shop. She could not believe it. She had not given permission. Why were they insisting on moving her mother to MNT Nursing Home without her permission? She stared at the wall in front of her thinking...you cannot do this! Is this their process? Can Stacey arrange the transfer without input or consent from family?

"I do not agree with her being transferred to MNT Nursing Home."

Phone signal at the lower level of the museum was poor. She was unable to hear a response from Stacey. Then, the call dropped. She stood there for a few minutes trying to figure out what to do next. She wondered, *so they do not give choices of facilities? And do they transfer patients who are having medical problems to other facilities that are not prepared to take care of them? This is too much.* Focusing on the museum right now is not possible for me, she reasoned. She thought for a moment—no response yet from their administration? Worried and nervous, Mara hurried back into the gift shop to find her father and brother. She found them near the baseball caps, trying to find the right cap for each. As she got closer to them, her dad said, "Is everything alright, sweetheart?"

Mara sighed with frustration and said to him, "No dad. That was the social worker at the facility, saying that they are transferring mummy to the same facility I told them that I do not want her to go to. I am sorry but I need to go to Baltimore."

Her father gave her a hug and said, "It is okay. We can go to see your mom." He placed the cap back on the rack and they exited the gift shop. They took the stairs to the first floor and left the museum to head to Baltimore.

She had to find the underlying cause of this. What was going on? Would she find one day that her mother had been transferred to a facility she had not approved? She called the insurance case manager, Toni.

"I heard that my mother was authorized to go to MNT Nursing Home, and I am not agreeing to that."

Toni sounded surprised, "Oh! Stacey at the Baltimore facility said that you had selected MNT Nursing Home."

Annoyed and disgusted by all this, Mara shook her head and told Toni, "I have never said that. I do not want my mother to go to MNT Nursing Home."

They ended the call when Toni said, "Okay. Point taken. I will just wait to know which facility you select. Take care. Bye."

Relieved that she had made Toni aware of her plans, Mara said "Okay thank you. Bye."

***

Mara's mind was focused on the Baltimore facility. And the floodgates busted open on her thoughts.

"Okay. So, their care is sub-standard, their customer service skills are awful, they do not seem to really feel for their patients. Why are they operating? Is it only me? Aren't other people complaining? Does this have something to do with "long-term acute care" not being really that? I almost begin to wish I were an investigator so I could compare. What is happening in other facilities? They are ignoring my wishes. I

do not understand why no matter how much I have empha-sized that I was not presented with choices of places for my mother to be transferred to, no one called or talked about al-ternatives with me. Are we stuck dealing with this facility because there is not much to choose from? Are they operating based on knowledge that patients and their families do not have other choices and simply must endure whatever is deliv-ered to them?"

Mara reasoned, "*some families may also have thought that as a health care establishment, the long-term acute care facility would be trustworthy.*" She continued to think things through.

"*My concern about advocating for my mother is retaliation. I wonder if other families have the same concerns. The problem is that I cannot just stay quiet and let things happen to my mother.*"

***

When Mara, Malcolm, and their father reached her mother's room, they noticed that her face was even more swollen. Mara asked her moth-er's nurse to speak with the intensivist. After several minutes, she heard Dr. Nabin's voice outside of the room. Mara, thinking quietly to herself, "*She is on again? She was here all last week.*"

Just seconds before she entered, Mara over-heard Dr. Nabin comment to the nurse at the pod table, "what does she want? I just spoke to her."

The thoughts came rushing in again. *"That's not accurate"* Mara thought. *"So they are talking about me. When did she "just speak" to me? They did not tell me they planned to move her. If they had told me, I would have been here and not at the museum. I cannot do this! Why are they making it so hard? Well, you can say whatever you like about me. Just remember that my mother is a patient. While unkind words cannot kill me, improper care could kill my mother. My job here is to advocate for my mother. I imagine that if you all cared about your mothers, you would do the same."*

Dr. Nabin entered the room with a smile on her face. "The edema was not as severe yesterday," Mara informed the physician. "I notice that her face is even more swollen today. I do not think that she is medically stable for discharge. The other issue is that my mom is complaining of abdominal pain. I am concerned because the level of care that she is to receive here is higher than at the subacute rehabilitation facility where she will transfer."

Dr. Nabin listened to Mara with a blank expression on her face. Mara continued, "The other issue is that I am familiar with the discharge process. I was not presented with a choice of facilities. I spoke with Stacey, the social worker and I told her that I would not give permission for my mother to be transferred to MNT Nursing Home."

Mara wondered if the discharge planning team had some sort of relationship with MNT that they kept insisting that her mother should transfer to that facility. Did they owe MNT Nursing Home something? Were they using the family to pay up debt?

Dr. Nabin said curtly, "I would decrease the rate on the feeding tube to see if that helps with the abdominal pain and perhaps adjust the dosage on the Lasix again."

Mara sensing the frustration from Dr. Nabin, wondered why were they making it so obvious that they wanted her mother out of their facility? She just wanted her mother to be okay. Shouldn't they be glad that there is a family member who wants to collaborate with the team? This was a family who did not just visit Denise, but one who addressed her needs. Mara and Denise's friend Breana were the visitors who provided personal care to Denise. This was not the family who visited and called constantly for staff to attend to Denise in ways that they themselves were able to assist. Mara and Breana were the ones who personally cleaned her when they visited and did not allow her to sit or lie in her wastes until a nursing assistant or nurse responded to their call several minutes later. They were the ones who would ask for supplies if none were available in the room and provide a total bath to Denise. Mara smiled as she quietly thought about the small acts of care and love from the family and friends.

"*But it also relieves staff of having one more patient to provide personal care to.*" She thought to herself. "*They are being compensated for services that mummy relies on them to provide, yet some of them seem to have no interest in doing so. Is this facility capable of providing the care that mummy needs? Or can they transfer her to a higher level of care? I asked the social worker to send my mother's clinical documentation to another long-term acute care hospital but admissions from the other facility told me that they never received it. I wonder what happened. How can I ensure that my mother receives proper care? Whenever I advocate and they listen, I notice the improvements in her health—she is not constantly sleepy from narcotics, the swelling in her face and arms decreased and she has less stomach pain. My hope is not to simply prolong her life, but it is to see her improve.*"

Thinking back about the conversation with the admissions liaison Maribeth, Mara wondered, "*Are they more concerned about length of stay? Are they also concerned that the health insurance would not pay for a stay beyond the three weeks? Would they keep patients like my mother at this facility with so many complications? Or do they consider transferring patients like her out to other facilities that may have a different approach with care? I just want her to get appropriate care, wherever she is.*"

***

Mara, her father, and brother visited with Denise for a couple of hours. Denise was tired. They knew that she was aware of their presence when she opened her eyes a few times, smiled and went back to sleep. They encouraged her to rest. She coughed a few times and Mara believed that she needed to be suctioned. She pressed the call bell and fifteen minutes went by without a nurse or nursing assistant responding.

Malcolm then went out to the nursing station and the nursing assistant at the desk told him that someone would be there. The wait after he returned to the room was even longer. While Mara and her family realized that Denise was not the only patient on the unit and that the staff may be busy with other patients, Denise was sick and required more attention than was being provided to her. While they continued to sit at her bedside, Denise's friend, Andrina, entered the room. Denise became more awake and smiled as her friend made silly jokes to get her to smile. They stayed a while longer. Mara prayed at her mother's side. Eventually a nurse walked in. She suctioned Denise.

"Are you okay?" She asked.

Denise nodded, then the nurse left the room. They wished Denise a good evening and left.

Mara visited again the next day. Now she trusted the facility even less than before. She had to be sure they did not do something she did not want done—like suddenly move her mother. Dr. Dhar, a pulmonologist whom Mara had not met before, walked into the room. He introduced himself to Denise and to Mara. He was of average build, in his mid-forties, of South Asian descent. He had a very pleasant smile, one that seemed genuine, not forced. He told Denise, "I am very pleased to see you sitting up in the chair."

She nodded and smiled, as if she had gone to the chair willingly. He was not present for the usual drama, whereby she had to be coaxed to transfer to the chair. He told her, "Your lab results look good, but I notice that you are having blood pressure issues. Your blood pressure is high." He asked, "Do you have any concerns?" His gaze shifted from mother to daughter and back to mother. Denise looked at Mara, knowing that her daughter would express her concerns and as if to say, "go ahead, tell him."

Mara told Dr. Dhar about her conversation with Dr. Bandara, the other pulmonologist, "I understand that my mother will not continue weaning here at this facility, according to Dr. Bandara. I absolutely disagree because I do not believe that my mom had a fair chance at the weaning. She was sick when she was being weaned from the ventilator. I told her that I am aware that my mom had fluid overload and pseudomonas at times when weaning was attempted. I am really asking you to reconsider." Mara suspected that Dr. Dhar had already known about her

conversation with his colleague; however, he provided no indication that he was aware of her conversation with the other doctor. The physician stood next
to Mara and listened.

"My mother was not strong enough when
she had pseudomonas and fluid overload during the
weaning trials."

Dr. Dhar did not openly express any dis-
agreement with his colleague, but he acknowledged
Mara's concerns by nodding and stated, "I was not
aware that the weaning trials were being done at
those times."

"I am in communication with the case
manager at the insurance company," Mara said.

At that point, the physician raised his eyebrows but said nothing.

Mara expressed, "I understand that there is
some concern on the facility's part that my mother's
stay would not be covered by the insurance company, but I was reassured that my mother continues to
meet criteria to be here and to receive the care for
which she was admitted."

Mara realized that most of what she told
Dr. Dhar, she had already communicated with someone else—Dr. Bandara, as well as administration
in her letter. She started to get tired of hearing
herself saying the same things but hoped

that the information would reach the right ears. She felt that desperate times called for desperate measures.

"I need to review the chart more closely and would write orders as I see appropriate." Dr. Dhar said, after a moment of silence. "Do you have any other questions or concerns?"

There were none.

"Take care. Have a good day," he said, before exiting the room. Soon after, Dr. Nabin entered.

"Does she not get any days off?" Mara wondered. "If she doesn't, that would explain why important aspects of my mother's care are being ignored and why it is obvious to me that she is irritated."

Dr. Nabin told Denise, "I am happy to see you in the chair!" Once again Denise smiled. Dr. Nabin examined Denise. She asked, "Any questions?"

Although it was not a question, Mara's concern was her mother's high blood pressure and she felt that it was necessary to communicate that to her. She told the physician, "I am really concerned about her elevated blood pressure and the fact that it impacts the therapy sessions. The physical and occupational therapists would not work with her because their protocol is to put therapy on hold if the vital signs are unstable and they do not think it is safe."

Mara would not encourage them to practice anything other than safety with her mother. She vowed not to be surprised by anything but found that she failed miserably in terms of the care that was provided to her mother. She was astonished to hear Dr. Nabin say, "Well I was unaware that her blood pressure has been elevated to the point that she is missing therapy."

To Mara's knowledge, the therapists had not worked with her mother for at least three sessions. Mara tried to process things in her mind — Somehow the pulmonologist who is new to mummy is aware of the elevated blood pressure, but the intensivist who has been involved all along, was not aware that there continued to be a problem with my mother's blood pressure. Dr. Nabin also told Mara, "She is deconditioned" with what to Mara seemed like an expression that said, 'so what do you want us to do?'

It was like night and day between that intensivist with whom she was speaking and the pulmonologist who had left the room minutes earlier. Mara tried to understand why they admitted her here? She is not receiving physical and occupational therapy and is not being weaned from the ventilator. The long-term acute care hospital uses an electronic system for documentation. In fact, it is the same application that was used at her hospital. Communication among providers regarding patient care would be easily accessible to the team if the resources were utilized.

Mara continued to speak with the physician, "She still has the mitten, and I do not understand the purpose. She has been itching for some time now and just needs some relief. She is also banging on the rails because she is uncomfortable and frustrated. With all due respect, if you were experiencing itching and could not verbally communicate with others, you would also want to have a way to be relieved."

It was an awkward moment, but she felt she had to make the analogy to get Dr. Nabin to think about it. Her mother was still under Dr. Nabin's care, and she remained hopeful that her mother would receive proper care.

She reminded Dr. Nabin, "She only has use of the right hand and it must be torturous for her to not have control of it."

After summarizing all of Mara's concerns in her mind, Dr. Nabin responded, "I'll add an as needed blood pressure medication and I'll discontinue the order for the mitten."

Mara was grateful. She said, "Thank you." Mara explained to her mother, "Mummy, try not to scratch here okay" as she pointed to the area on her mother's chest where the dialysis catheter was removed. She told her mother, "Perhaps if you just tap it, you may get some relief, but it would also indicate to the staff that you're itching and they would hopefully apply some lotion." Denise nodded as she mouthed the word, "Okay."

***

Denise was not a difficult patient and Mara was her voice. It was possible that some of the staff did not have a good understanding or any knowledge of her medical history. Mara wondered whether they did their own assessments. They relied primarily on the information that was sent to them by the Northern Metropolitan Hospital; even from there significant medical information had been withheld. The information that seemed to have made its way to the facility was the fact that Denise's daughter was an advocate for her mother and that she wanted her to thrive. Perhaps the information that they received from the Northern Metropolitan Hospital was more of a warning about Denise's daughter and that she was a difficult family member. Mara thought, there are a few nurses, nursing assistants and respiratory therapists who provide care appropriately and treat her mother with care and respect. They are in a minority here. They treat visitors with respect. They are not defensive. They functioned appropriately in their various roles. They were not simply performing tasks. Mara believed they seemed to be genuinely concerned about her mother. They were professional and introduced themselves when they entered the room and her mother appeared to be comfortable with them.

There were times that Denise told Mara whom she thought was nice. She was sufficiently aware to know how she was being treated and to react to the treatment. One evening, Dana slowly walked into Denise's room.

"Ms. Mitchell, I hope you have a nice evening," she said. "I am off tomorrow. I will see you when I get back."

Denise smiled. Dana walked out of the room. Denise looked over at her daughter, she motioned her head toward Dana and smiled. She mouthed, "she's nice."

Not long after, Gail and Greg, the respiratory therapists walked in the room. They were doing their bedside report.

Greg asked, "How are you doing?"

Denise mouthed, "I'm okay." Greg smiled.

The therapists slowly walked out of the room. Denise looked over at Mara and gave a thumbs up.

Chapter 25

You're speaking!

What a difference five and a half months makes since the angioedema! Denise was now tolerating sitting up in the chair for longer periods. Her friend Cathy who worked in Baltimore visited her during her lunch breaks. Denise loved that.

Sometimes, Cathy visited after work with one or both of her daughters. One day, when Mara was at work, her Aunt Cathy called her on facetime so that Denise could see her.

"Mar, I am with mom. She is coming along well," Aunt Cathy said.

Mara quickly walked down the hallway to the visitors' waiting area. She could see her mother on the screen. They both smiled. Mara said, "Thanks Auntie Cathy! Hi mummy. You are doing really well. I am so glad to see your face. I will see you this evening after work."

Denise nodded. She started to cough. The respiratory therapist was in the room. She suctioned Denise. Auntie Cathy moved the phone away from Denise. She and Mara kept smiling at each other.

"Mom is getting there," Auntie Cathy said. "She just needs more time. Mar, I got to run but we will chat later." They ended their call.

Another time, the speech therapist was present, and Mara asked her over the phone about her mother's progress. The speech therapist told Mara, "We are trying to work with her using the speaking valve. She is not ready for it, yet it seems." Mara said, "Okay thanks. She will get there." Once when Auntie Cathy called, they were attempting to have Denise use the speaking valve again. Mara could see her mother trying to speak but could not hear her.

One day, when Mara picked up the phone. It was a facetime call. She was surprised to hear her mother's voice. She stared at the screen to make sure it was her mother speaking. Mara opened her eyes wide, then her mouth opened and remained opened for a few seconds. She smiled. Denise had a smile on her face and as she looked at her daughter on the screen, she said "Mara, Mara, Mara" in what sounded as a very hoarse voice. Mara was grinning from ear to ear.

"Hi mummy! You are doing great!"

"Mara, I love you. I love you so much. Mara, I miss you," Denise said.

Then Denise started to cry—tears of joy, Mara was sure. She was in disbelief that she was hearing her mother's voice.

"I love you too mummy," Mara replied, still overjoyed by the moment. "You are doing so well. I will see you this evening after work. I am so proud of you. You are getting there."

As Mara looked out the window of the conference room, she thought, "She said she missed me! I visit her all the time, so I guess she means talking to me."

Within a few minutes, Denise started to cough and so the therapist decided to discontinue the speaking valve. She said that they would continue to try it during the next therapy session with her. Mara told her mother one more time, "I will see you this evening, mummy. Bye, bye."

Denise responded with a nod. She said "bye" and smiled.

Chapter 26

Roles and responsibility

Later that evening, when Mara went to visit, they were both extremely excited. Denise was lying in the bed with the head of the bed elevated. Mara walked to her mother's bedside and hugged her. They stayed embraced and smiled at each other.   "You're doing really well mummy," Mara said. Denise continued to smile. "You must keep trying. Excellent job. You are getting there."

Denise mouthed 'yes, thanks' and smiled the sweet way that she had always smiled.

"Okay mummy let us do some exercises. We can start with your right arm. Lift your right arm to point to the ceiling ten times."

Denise looked up at her daughter and began to lift her arm. They counted together. Denise mouthed 'one, two, three...she counted to ten.

"We'll work with your left arm together," Mara said.

As Mara tried to extend the fingers on her mother's left hand, her mother winced. She was clearly in pain. Mara paused. She rubbed her mother's hand. She tried again to extend her mother's fingers—this time slower. Denise folded in her bottom lip and bit down. She closed her eyes and turned her head to face the other side. "I am sorry mummy. Okay, I got it."

She stopped as she placed the rubber pencil that her mother's friend, Auntie Breana had brought to help prevent the fingers from being permanently deformed.

"You're okay?" Mara asked.

Denise nodded. "Let's continue" Mara said. "Can you lift your left arm?"

Denise looked at the arm and lifted it about an inch off the bed. Mara smiled. "Good" she said. She supported her mother's left arm and began to lift it up toward the ceiling. She kept looking at her mother. Denise's facial expression was relaxed. She did not appear to be in any more pain.

"Okay mummy let us work on the legs. Can you lift your left leg?" Denise looked down at her left leg. She lifted her left leg off the bed but was unable to support it for more than two lifts. Mara supported her mother's left knee and left ankle. She helped her mother to complete ten lifts.

"I know you can do the right leg," Mara said. "Lift the right leg ten times."

Denise smiled and lifted her right leg off the bed as she counted, 'one, two, three…' until she got to ten. The evening nurse walked into the room.

"Hello. I am Debra. I will be the nurse this evening," she said to Denise and to Mara. Denise smiled and mouthed "hello."

"Hi Debra. I was just working with my mom's left hand, and it is difficult to extend her fingers. She has a splint here on the table and the schedule is on the wall. Can you please remind the staff that they need to stick to the schedule? Whenever the splint is not used, her fingers become harder to extend."

Mara lifted the splint off the bedside table to show the nurse what she was referring to. Debra walked closer to the table to look at the splint. She looked at Mara, "Oh okay. Yes. I will pass this on in report. I am sorry."

Mara thought to herself, *okay this nurse seems to be understanding. It may be getting better now. I think they are getting the point. They seem more interested now. They are seeing progress because I have been pushing. But what about people whose family members do not know enough to advocate? This place worries me. Is this what always happens? Do you have to be knowledgeable to advocate? But I cannot worry about everyone now. I am glad this seems to be working. Lord, I hope I am right! I really do not want my mother's hand to be permanently deformed. Why would they just ignore it? Her hand was normal before she went into the hospital. I told the therapists this. Couldn't the therapists exercise her hand and make sure that the staff was following the schedule for the splint? Was this attitude normalized within the health system?*

Mara continued to monitor her mother's lab results and vital signs. She remained in close contact with her two aunts Ali and Simone and provided them with the information. As medical doctors, they asked the kinds of questions that doctors would ask. Auntie Ali wanted to know about the blood pressure and laboratory results. Auntie Simone asked about Denise's mental status.

Now, Denise started to experience abdominal cramping. Dr. Nabin attributed the cramping to diarrhea, but she said she was not sure. Mara inquired about the new tube feeding formula. She wondered whether that might explain the cramping. Her mother, she knew, was lactose intolerant. The facility would know that, too. Would they? Of course, they should. Again, she began to wonder. The nurses told her that it was not the tube feeding that caused the cramping. The lab results were improving and did not explain the cramping. Her potassium was slightly low but she had low potassium for a long time, even prior to being hospitalized. When Mara visited, she could see that her mother was extremely uncomfortable. The physician ordered that the nurses decrease the tube feeding rate but that did not seem to alleviate her discomfort. Her nurse gave her pain medication. She rested quietly until she fell asleep. Mara prayed at her mother's side.

"Lord, thank you for giving mummy the strength to get this far. Please protect her. Bless the caregivers and give them everything that they need to provide safe care to her. Lord, I know that all things are possible with you, and I am looking forward to seeing mummy back on her feet again. In Jesus name I pray. Amen."

She left soon after the end of visiting hours. She sent out messages as usual to ask people to continue to pray for her mother.

Meantime, other administrative things were happening. Mara received a response in the mail from the Baltimore Long Term Acute Care hospital about the letter that she had sent to administration.

***

June 12, 2017

Dear Ms. Mitchell,

Thank you for your letter regarding concerns with your mother's care at Baltimore Long

Term Acute Care Hospital. I apologize for the experience you described and take your concerns seriously. The team conducted an investigation based on the information you provided. The investigation was completed on June 9, 2017. It included a review of your mother's medical record and interviews with staff involved in her care.

I appreciate the thorough background of your mother's case. It was helpful for me to get your full perspective. Your mother started with the recover program on February 24. On April 28, your mother scored 20/23 on the JFK coma recovery scale. Following, your mother experienced some medical issues, and she was given an extra week for the recover program. Your mother did not achieve a score of 22/23, which was one of the criteria to continuing in the recover program. Barrier to achieving this score included continued restlessness, low frustration tolerance, anxiety, and inability to focus long enough to answer questions and follow commands. On May 12, your mother was seen for physical therapy interventions five times per week for two weeks. Your mother was reported to be at maximum assistance for bed mobility and for out of bed activities she required total assistance. Per documentation and speaking with staff involved in your mom's care, she is able to tolerate sitting out of bed for limited periods of time.

It is not uncommon for our patients to have some medical setbacks during the weaning and rehab process. Your mother's first weaning attempt was March 3 until March 8 per the weaning protocol. During that time, your mother developed increased shortness of breath and an increased white blood cell count associated with acute bacteremia and pneumonia. The second attempt for weaning began on March 17, which was ended that same day due to lethargy. Her third attempt was started on March 28 and ended on April 4 when she developed tachypnea and respiratory acidosis. At this time, your mother also developed increased renal issues. Her fourth weaning attempt was started on May 1. On May 2, she became tachypnetic, with increased respiratory acidosis. Your mother's cultures were positive for Pseudomonas, Klebsiellas and Stenotrophomonas. The fifth attempt at weaning was on May 9. On May 10, she had increased carbon dioxide levels with lethargy and desaturations and weaning was stopped.

I personally spoke with the attending physician on Monday May 22. At that time, we discussed your mother's case at length. It is true that some attempts were made under less than ideal conditions; several were made without these handicaps. However, I am pleased to know that it was decided that a sixth weaning attempt began on May 24. I understand that she is doing well and on trach collar trials during the day and CPAP at night. Thank you for allowing us another chance to be successful. The team is aiming for only vent support at night.

As you are aware, restraint orders may be applied in emergency situations or as the last resort in order to ensure the patient safety. Your mother displayed signs and symptoms of unsafe behaviors that were putting her at risk. When all attempts to address and redirect the unsafe behaviors were unsuccessful, the physician wrote and order for a temporary hand mitten. The hand mitten was discontinued shortly after.

I regret about your experience with the social work staff member. It is the expectation of all staff to provide the utmost customer service experience. The social worker should play a key role in advocating for patients and families. Our philosophy and approach to supporting families is to always be mindful of the patient and family experience and offer support. She was provided education and the concern was addressed by her director. In addition, our Manager of Respiratory Care, reviewed the concerns with the interaction between your mother and the Respiratory Therapist and appropriate action was taken.

Again, than[k] you for sharing your concerns and allowing us to investigate. The team at Baltimore Long Term Acute Care Hospital wishes the very best for your mother. We look forward to continuing to provide you the best quality care and experience while [s]he is patient at Baltimore Long Term Acute Care Hospital. I again extend my apologies for your experience. If you have any additional questions, please feel free to contact me at 410-000-0000.

Sincerely,

Vice President, Medical Affairs

Mara sighed. *"This letter is not entirely true. If I had not been at the bedside as often, I would not have had an argument. Their minds were made up about us before we arrived at this facility."*

Chapter 27

Feeling uncomfortable

Denise continued at the facility during June 2017. It was now seven months since that day when she had gone to the ER and had to be admitted. Mara felt proud and pleased when she looked at her mother these days. She was so clearly improving. Perhaps she wondered why her daughter sometimes looked at her and kept smiling. For Mara, watching her mother take it for granted that she could write or whisper something…was surreal.

One afternoon, Mara and two of Denise's close friends who were sisters, Audrea, and Haley, were visiting. Denise told them that there was a nurse whom she did not want to have care for her anymore because she did not feel comfortable with the care that he provided. She printed his name in her notepad. They asked her to explain what happened. She indicated by crossing her right arm over her chest to touch her left shoulder. She mouthed, "I didn't feel comfortable."

Of course, since communication was still not perfect after the strokes, she had difficulty explaining but she was clear about her discomfort. When Mara read the name of the nurse that her mother had written, she knew who he was. He always was kind in her presence. Could he be that kind of person? Of course, he could. He seemed professional in her presence, but who knows who people are? And her mother had been uncomfortable enough to share her reservations. They had to listen. As Denise described it by mouthing her words and with gestures, Manuel—the worker, lifted her head forward to fix the pillow behind her head; however, she felt uncomfortable with the way he held her against himself. Audrea requested to speak with the nursing supervisor. She wanted to report Denise's comments.

While they awaited the nursing supervisor, Denise's grandson's mother Natalie appeared. She waited with them, and they discussed Ean, Mara's nephew and Denise's grandson, who lived abroad with her. They were visiting for the summer. After several minutes of waiting, a tall, broad-shouldered man of African descent walked down the hallway toward them. He wore a white lab coat. He got closer, smiled briefly, and said, "Hello. Are you the Mitchell family?" He had a deep voice.

"Yes, we are," Audrea responded.

The gentleman held his clipboard with both hands a little lower than his stomach.

"I am James. The nursing supervisor," he said. He glanced around at all the faces looking at him. "How can I help you?"

"We all love Denise," Audrea responded. "She means a lot to us. We are concerned about some of the things that she has told us. There is a nurse that makes her uncomfortable. She does not want him to care for her anymore."

James remained standing with his legs apart. He had one hand crossed over the other on the clipboard. He looked directly at Audrea.

"I see. I will talk to Ms. Mitchell and the facility would investigate the report. I will see her now."

Mara, Audrea, Haley, and Natalie followed him to Denise's room. He walked straight to Denise's bedside.

"Ms. Mitchell. I am James, the nursing supervisor. I need to talk to you about the complaint that you made to your family. Can you tell me what happened?"

Denise looked up at him. She nodded. She began to mouth what happened. There was no sound. James tried to read her lips but could not.

He said, "nurse?" Denise nodded. She picked up her clipboard and printed the name Manuel. She attempted to write more but just wrote Manuel's name again.

"He did something?" James said.

She nodded.

"What did he do?"

Denise gestured by placing her right arm across her chest to touch her left shoulder, while she continued to mouth her report.

"Okay," James said. "He did something and you were uncomfortable?"

Denise nodded and mouthed, "yes."

"The nurse manager will come to see you on Monday. The facility will investigate. Thanks for your time, Ms. Mitchell." She responded by mouthing, "thank you."

As he walked away from the bed, he looked at Denise's family and said, "Okay. Thank you. Bye."

No one said anything else in the room about the incident. Mara thought quietly to herself—*Not even an apology to her that she felt uncomfortable? Maybe that's the facility's policy.*

***

Two days after her mother's complaint, Mara was sitting at her desk at work when she received a phone call from the facility's customer relations person, Debra.

"The facility is conducting an investigation about your mom's complaint," she told Mara. "The facility needs about fourteen days from the initial report before we can provide an outcome."

Mara listened quietly and responded, "okay thank you Debra."

It wasn't clear to Mara how they conducted their investigation, and she didn't see Manuel again when she visited the facility.

There had already been an issue with slow response to the call bell whenever any of Denise's visitors, including Mara, called for assistance. After the report that resulted in Manuel being prohibited from caring for Denise, the response time from staff worsened. Were they short staffed? Or was this punishment? Were they saying she should not have complained? Were they signaling that they did not believe her? Did they think that she, Mara, had made the complaint? If she is not comfortable with him, whether he's doing something, he knows he should be ashamed of, she's just not comfortable with him! Mara sighed. Never a dull moment.

Chapter 28

Slow weaning

It was now the beginning of July 2017. In the fifth month of Denise's stay at the Baltimore facility, the struggle continued. Now, they were focusing on again trying to wean her from the ventilator so that she would be able to breathe fully on her own.

The respiratory therapists followed orders for a slow weaning process. One evening, Mara was at her mother's bedside when one of the respiratory therapists, Megan, was attending to her. Megan placed her hand on Denise's left shoulder and as she looked down at her, she told her, "You are doing well, Ms. Mitchell. You have come a long way."
Denise smiled. Megan looked over at Mara who was sitting on the chair next to the bed. She said to Mara, "You know she's on trach collar for twelve hours and is back on the vent at night." Mara opened her eyes wide and smiled. "Really?" Mara said.

Megan smiled too. She said, "Yes. Sometimes she stays on trach collar longer." She looked down at Denise and said, "Just keep going. You are doing great."

Denise smiled and nodded. Mara pictured her mother being on trach collar only, without being connected to the ventilator. The humidified oxygen would be given through the tracheostomy on her mother's neck. She imagined that soon her mother would be free from the ventilator and would receive oxygen through the tracheostomy. Denise looked over at Mara and continued to smile.

***

Mara continued to call daily from her job to receive updates from her mother's nurse or physician. Vital signs were stable. She was making strides with the weaning. Mara drove to the Baltimore facility every evening to make sure that her mother knew that she was still there, that she was supporting her. It was difficult for Denise's colleagues and other friends to visit regularly as the facility was a bit far from everyone. Mara was uncertain as to whether her mother knew when her friend Grace from her job had visited. Denise was happy to show her a drawing that was made by Grace's young daughter. The drawing was on the wall in front of Denise's bed. She pointed toward it and mouthed, "Grace's daughter." She was coming along. Mara continued to send out daily text messages to family and friends:

Hello everyone, mummy is tolerating being off the vent for more hours, up to twelve for two consecutive days. She will soon be transferred to a subacute rehab facility, after it is determined that there are no other medical issues that need to be addressed. I will update once she is ready for discharge. Thanks for the continued prayers and support.

As the slow weaning continued, Mara remained in contact with the insurance case manager, Toni, to ensure that her mother still had insurance coverage at the facility. Toni confirmed continued authorization. Denise became more alert but was still not receiving therapy services due to her 'anxiety'. Mara assessed that they were truly making preparations for her to live at a nursing home. They did not really seem to think they could work toward her living at home on her own. They are wrong! They are too quick to ascribe things to anxiety and not to their way of doing things. Her mother was no longer on full ventilator support but was now able to tolerate as many as fifteen hours of being on the trach collar and then back on the ventilator at night. This was exciting for Denise, her family, and friends. Mara and Auntie Myrna looked at each other and said, "Chalk and Cheese!" they laughed, realizing that not everybody who happened to hear the comment would realize that this was derived from an old English saying, signaling how different things were. And they were! Denise's situation today was vastly different from what it had been just a month before. She was on the road to recovery.

Mara spoke with Stacey, the social worker, again. They discussed other choices of facilities. Denise had to be transferred to a subacute rehabilitation facility also known as a skilled nursing facility that accepted patients on the ventilator and performed weaning. Mara's first choice based on the ratings and location was Lory Alden. That facility was located about half hour drive away from Mara's home. She was also interested in Lory in Columbia and her third choice was the Alexandria Nursing and Rehabilitation Center. There were not many options to select from based on Denise's needs. She required a facility that provided ventilator weaning that was in-network with her health insurance. Proximity to Mara's home was also a key factor. Although there were not many options to select from, it turned out that MNT Nursing Home was not the only vent-weaning skilled nursing facility in the Washington D.C. metropolitan area, as the Baltimore facility must have believed—or must have wanted to believe. There were a few others. Auntie Breana and Mara toured Lory Alden and were pleased with the facility based on their tour. Denise was accepted. They had not toured the facility in

Alexandria together due to Mara's schedule and she was certain that her mother would transfer to Lory Alden.

But sometimes the best of plans does not work out. Unfortunately, when Denise was again deemed medically stable for discharge, Lory Alden was not able to accept her, as there were no beds available at the time. Since there was an accepting facility that the insurance would cover, Mara had no choice but to allow the transfer to the Alexandria facility. If Denise did not transfer to the accepting facility because of Mara waiting for a bed to become available at Lory Alden, based on her understanding of the discharge planning process, Mara knew that she would have been billed for her mother's continued stay at the Baltimore facility. She would have received a denial letter from the insurance company, a medical necessity denial letter for continued stay at the Baltimore facility. Mara did not have any more discussions with the facility about her mother's need to continue to stay. In fact, from their behavior, it was evident that they wanted Denise to be transferred out, and Mara preferred to have her mother transfer out safely without any more issues. Her hope was that her mother was not now making a transition that would feel like she was jumping out of the frying pan and into the fire.

Chapter 29

Plan to transfer from LTACH to subacute rehabilitation facility

On July 7, 2017, the day of the actual transfer, Mara received a call from Stacey who informed her of the time that the ambulance would pick up her mother from the Baltimore facility to transport her to Alexandria.

"The ambulance is scheduled to pick up your mom at 3:30pm today to take her to the Alexandria rehab. I would suggest that rather than you driving to Baltimore, you can meet her at the Alexandria facility. She should arrive by approximately 5pm, considering traffic. The discharge paperwork has all the information that the Alexandria rehab needs. Okay."

Mara listened quietly to Stacey and just as the call was about to end, Stacey remarked, "I'm not optimistic that your mother will get off the vent."

What? She did not know that Denise was only on the ventilator at night at that point. During the daytime, Denise received her oxygen via the tracheostomy. Why would Stacey say a thing like that?

"As her daughter, as a nurse, as a Christian, it's God I put my trust in," Mara responded.

Mara arrived at the Alexandria facility at approximately 4:25pm on the afternoon of her mother's scheduled transfer. She waited in the dining room where the ladies at the nursing station had instructed her to wait. After about 20 minutes, one of the nurses asked her, "Are you waiting for Mitchell?" She responded yes.

"She was transferred to Simion Hospital," The nurse told her.

"What? Do you know what happened?"

"No. They just said she is not coming today. She was transferred to the hospital."

Mara immediately called Stacey but there was no response. She left a voicemail message requesting a return call. She was about to go upstairs to speak to the admissions' liaison, Veronica, when she decided to call instead, "Hi Veronica. This is Mara, Denise's daughter. I am here at the rehab and was just told that my mom was transferred to Simion hospital. Do you know what happened?"

Veronica, who sounded surprised to hear from Mara said, "Mara. I'm so sorry. I do not know what happened to your mom. I did not call you because I just assumed that Stacey would have called you. It was Stacey who called to inform me that your mom was transferred to Simion Hospital." Puzzled, Mara said, "Okay. Thanks Veronica." Stacey did not call. Mara whispered to herself, "God does not like ugly."

Mara stood looking around her, thinking about driving to Baltimore. *How far away is that from here? I am sure it is more than an hour. It is rush hour so it will be longer.*

***

Simion Hospital

Mara was still on the lower level of the Alexandria Rehab. She wondered about what to do next. She hurried to the elevator. She sighed, "It is 4:55pm. Traffic will be horrible. It is rush-hour. Everyone is at work or getting off from work. Who can I ask to go with me to Baltimore now?"

The elevator doors opened. She walked out quickly and pulled her car key out of her bag. She walked out of the front door. Her car was parked across from the entrance of the building. She got in and sat there for a moment. She continued to think, "Okay. I need to use Waze for directions. I have no idea how to get there from here. She put on Waze.

Who can I call? I do not know who I can call to drive all the way to Baltimore with such short notice. I doubt anyone would want to go. I really wish I had a partner that I could call."

She googled the phone number to Simion hospital. She dialed. "Operator" said a woman on the other end.

"Hi operator," Mara responded. "My mother Denise Mitchell was admitted there this afternoon. Can you transfer me to her nurse or doctor please?"

"Sure, hold the line."

She waited for someone to come on the line. Someone else was calling her. She could see the number. It looks like a number from the same hospital. Should she put this call on hold? Would she miss an important call? Quickly she ended the call and accepted the other one.

"Hello" she said. "Is this Ms. Mara Mitchell?"

Mara breathed heavily, "yes, it is." The male voice on the other end said, "Hi. I'm Dr. Matthews at Simion Hospital. Your mother came into the emergency room by ambulance this afternoon. She lost consciousness and did not have a pulse in the ambulance as she was being transported to the Alexandria rehabilitation facility.

The paramedics had performed CPR and her pulse returned and she regained consciousness. As a result of this incident, she was admitted to the intensive care unit here at Simon Hospital and would remain on the ventilator. We will monitor her closely."

"Okay. Thank you, Dr. Matthews. I am on my way there."

"See you then. Bye."

***

So! That is what happened. Why would that happen again? Still, I am glad she regained consciousness. Oh goodness! Traffic is so heavy. Oh mummy, I really need you to be okay. You have come a long way. I keep telling you to look away from the light when you are unconscious, and a light is calling you to some other place. Look away from the light!

Mara began to cry. She continued to speak out aloud. "There is always something. Why? Dear Lord. You have gotten mummy this far. Please protect her. Please bless the people who are taking care of her. Guide them and help them to make the best decisions. Keep mummy safe. Please Lord." Mara sighed, "I will just update everyone after I get to Baltimore. This is way too much for one person. Ughh! Way too much!"

She arrived at the Baltimore hospital to which her mother had been transferred.

Simion, she realized, was directly across the street from the long-term acute care hospital. Mara arrived on the unit a few minutes before 7pm. The security guard at the front desk told her that she would have to wait until 8pm. Visitors were not allowed between 6:30pm - 8pm. Mara sat on the chair in the waiting room across from him, leaned her head back and closed her eyes.

"I will not send out an update yet until I see her and know that she is okay. I should let Auntie Myrna know."

She dialed, "Hi. Auntie Myrna. Mummy was transferred to Simion Hospital in Baltimore this afternoon. She lost consciousness in the ambulance and was transferred here. I am waiting to see her." Her aunt Myrna sounded alarmed, "Oh no! Is she okay?"

Mara folded her lips, "The doctor said she is. I have to wait until 8 o'clock to see her."

"I'm sorry Mara," Myrna said. "Try not to worry. Call me when you know something."

Mara rubbed the back of her neck, "Thanks Auntie Myrna. Bye."

What a day! First, she had driven thirty-five miles from Germantown, Maryland, expecting to see her mother at the rehab in Alexandria, Virginia. She had then driven another fifty-nine miles from Alexandria to Baltimore, Maryland to see her mother there, at Simion Hospital. She looked at her phone and realized that she had received a few messages, requesting updates on her mom. *Ok. I may as well just update people now.* She sat in the waiting room and sent out messages:

Mummy was on her way to Alexandria Rehab and had some sort of trouble. She was admitted to Simion Hospital. I am waiting to see her.

***

At 8pm, the guard said to her and others waiting that they could go in to visit. She hurried behind the other male guard who opened the door for them to come in. He stopped in front of room 6 and turned to Mara, "This is it." The glass doors to her mother's room were closed. Mara could see a nurse at the bedside. The nurse saw Mara as well. She came to the door.

"Hi. Can you give me a few minutes?" She smiled.

"Sure…" Mara forcing a small smile.

A few minutes later, the nurse came to the door, "Miss, you may come in now."

Denise was wide awake. She seemed eager to talk to Mara, "They said that I lost consciousness."

Her face crumpled and she started to cry. Mara leaned her head on her mother's head and placed her arm around her.

"It is okay mummy. You are going to be okay." Although Denise had only been there for about two hours, she told Mara, "It's a different caliber of people." Mara laughed.

"Well, how you know that already, Mummy?"

"But it is true. You could tell."

There was a knock on the glass door. Mara turned. It was the nurse who had just left the room.

"I am Kaley. I'll be her nurse tonight. Can I just verify that we have your phone number, correct?" She read the phone number from the chart.

"Yes. It's correct," Mara smiled.

"I will be right out here. If you have any questions, please feel free to ask."

A few minutes later, a tall slender man wearing a white lab coat walked into the room.

"Hi, I am Dr. Matthews. I believe we spoke. Are you, her daughter?"

"Yes, I am Mara."

"It looks like the reason she lost consciousness was a mucus plug. We will keep an eye on her here in the ICU. Do you have any questions?"

"No. Nothing, I can think of right now. Thank you."

"Alright. Let us know if you do. Take care." He walked out of the room.

Denise remained at Simion Hospital for three days. She was stable in the ICU with no issues. The staff was very polite and professional. Her only grandson, Ean, was visiting from abroad with his mother. The security guard was kind enough to allow Ean to enter the ICU. It was a concession because Ean was 9 years old and there were age restrictions for visitors. Denise was extremely happy to see him. She smiled and stared at him, as if she did not believe that he was there. She touched his face and smiled her infectious smile. Mara was also incredibly happy to see her nephew and was grateful that his mother had brought him to brighten her mother's day. They took pictures. Mara knew that her mother had trouble with her short-term memory given all that she had been through. She planned to show her mother the pictures that she had taken with her grandson later.

Denise spent about a day and a half in the ICU and was transferred to the intermediate care unit. Mara watched the staff as they walked in and out of her mother's room. She thought to herself, "Wow. They are so patient and kind here. Such a vast difference in care, just across the street. So, it is not me. I am doing the same thing I did over there. Everyone is professional and receptive to information about mummy."

They seemed to think what Mara would have expected—that more information allowed them to provide care appropriately. They put Denise back on full ventilator support. Both Denise and Mara were disappointed that she was placed back on the ventilator, but they understood.

"Mummy, this is temporary okay."

"I know," Denise said. "I just want to go home." Her voice could be heard clearly as she had support from the ventilator.

The social worker at the hospital, Arlene, contacted Mara by phone. Mara told her, "My mom was being transferred to the Alexandria rehab from the Baltimore Long Term Acute Care hospital for short term rehab and to wean from the ventilator."

Arlene replied, "Okay. Good to know. I may have to obtain authorization again from the insurance for the Alexandria rehab, as well as, for the ambulance."

She gave that explanation because she was unaware of how much time it would take to obtain the authorization. Mara appreciated Arlene's honesty and interest in preparing her for any obstacles related to the transfer. Denise was ready for discharge and the authorizations were obtained for both transportation and the rehabilitation center. Mara thought to herself, "Arlene is truly kind and professional. She sounds as though she was well-trained and demonstrates empathy."

This experience made Mara smile and remembered her training. "Good! So, people were really being trained. This felt good. It should never be an unusual experience when people, especially trained caregivers, showed kindness. Okay. So we had to have this experience at Simion hospital to remind us that good-natured people exist, and that the health-care system works well in some places."

It was hard to have to do this, but ... who knows why?"

Chapter 30

Transfer to Alexandria rehab

On July 11, 2017, at last, Denise arrived at the Alexandria Nursing and Rehabilitation Center. The facility is located in downtown Alexandria, Virginia, in a residential neighborhood. Denise was certainly crisscrossing the DMV—D.C., Maryland, and Virginia for care. The Alexandria facility is easily accessible via Metro for train riders. It is also close to the 395 highway. As she drove on the highway, Mara began to think about the commute. *This place is easy to get to. The problem with it is there is a lot of traffic.* As she got onto the main street after getting off the highway, she looked for the building. She remembered driving there a few days prior. It was off the main road on a little hill. It was an older brick building.

Mara was anxious about the transfer and prayed that her mother would have a smooth transition to the rehab. She stood in the hallway on the unit to which her mother was being transferred, so that they could see each other when she arrived.

Denise saw her daughter standing in the hallway and immediately started to indicate with her hand that she wanted her to come in the room. One of the nurses told her, "Your daughter can come in when we are done with the assessment."

Mara leaned against the wall outside of her mother's room. *My goodness. This assessment process is quite lengthy. They keep going in and out of the room. I am guessing these are nurses and nursing assistants. Why do they have to keep going in and out so much?* Usually, the assessment would be a complete body examination. The staff would examine Denise's skin and document their findings, such as whether she had any pressure ulcers, any rashes, or any finding on her skin. They would complete that examination as a baseline for her condition upon arrival to their facility. What else would be included in their assessment? Would there be anything more?

"Ms. Mitchell, you may come in now."

Denise smiled when she saw her. She casually passed her right hand across her face as if she were making herself presentable. She was sitting upright on the bed. She was wearing a hospital gown. As she entered the room, Mara noticed the restroom to the left. Outside of it, there was a sink. Straight ahead, on entering the room, she saw the large window that spanned the length of the room. At the foot of the bed was a dresser and a closet. There were two nightstands on each side of the bed. On top of the nightstand to the left side, sat a small ventilator. On the other nightstand, there were some respiratory supplies.

Denise was on full ventilator support again. Her voice was audible. She introduced Mara to her nurse, "Mara this is my nurse Ann. This is my daughter."

For a moment, Mara did not think of her mother as a patient. *She is feeling well enough to make introductions!* She was her usual self in that conversation. The nurse Ann, perhaps West African, had a serious expression, but she smiled and nodded during the introductions.

"This is the Respiratory unit" Ann said as she pointed toward the floor. She continued to speak as she moved both hands around, "If you need anything Ms. Mitchell, press the red button. I am not sure about visiting hours because the facility has been flexible with visiting hours. Do you have any questions?" She looked at Denise and then at Mara.

"No," Denise responded.

Mara smiled at Ann, "Thank you. No, I do not have any questions."

Well, I have to ask someone else about the visiting hours. I must pass that information to other people who may want to come to visit. I do not want to be reprimanded again for violating visiting hours. Anyway, that is the least of my concerns right now.

A female voice came on the overhead intercom. Mara listened. Oh, it is about visiting hours. She looked at her phone and saw the time, 8pm. The female voice announced, "Attention all visitors, visiting hours have ended. Please use the side doors on the first floor to exit the building. Thank you for your cooperation. Have a good evening."

Mara opened her mouth as though surprised, "Mummy, there was a very pleasant lady at the desk who welcomed me earlier and now she is directing me on how to leave the building." Denise laughed and then started to cough. The small ventilator in the room alarmed so loudly when she coughed that it startled both. There seemed to be a vast difference between the equipment here and similar equipment at the long-term acute care hospital and the ones at the acute care hospital. The ventilator at the hospitals in Baltimore and in Northern Montgomery County were large machines that sat on the floor. At this nursing facility, it was a small loud machine that sat on the nightstand.

Mara realized that because Denise was on isolation for an infection, she had been given a private room at the far end of the hallway. Wasn't this a bit far from the nursing station? That machine was loud enough, though. They could hear it from anywhere on the unit. The nurse, Ann, walked into the room.

"Are you okay?" She asked Denise. Denise smiled and affirmed with a nod that she was okay.
"Oh! Such a beautiful smile."

Mara smiled too, "Ann here's my number if you need it, 571-000-0000." Ann wrote the number on her clipboard.

"Okay, thank you. Have a good night," she said to Mara. Ann walked out of the room.

Mara stood next to her mother's bed, mentally preparing herself for goodbyes.

"Okay mummy let us pray. Lord thank you for all that you have done. Thank you for all that you continue to do. Mummy has gotten this far. We know that all things are possible with you, and we are asking you to give her the strength to continue toward a full recovery. We ask that you bless the caregivers and give them everything that they need to provide safe care to her. In Jesus name we pray. Amen." She hugged and kissed her mother. Denise looked up at her, "get home safe." As she walked down the hallway, Mara saw a few nurses at the nursing station.

"Goodnight," she said.

They responded, "goodnight."

It was good that they responded. She got to her car, "I really hope she will be okay in this place. This is beginning to feel so routine. Help her, Lord!"

She drove home—out on to the main road, to Interstate 395N to 495 and then along I270N. It took her 40 minutes to get home to the edges of Montgomery County, Maryland. As soon as she got in her house, she wrote her text:

Hello everyone, mummy transferred this evening to the rehab to continue with the weaning and for therapy. Please feel free to visit her and provide support for continued progress. She is at the

Alexandria Rehabilitation Center

Thanks for the continued prayers and support.

***

The next morning while at work, Mara contacted the rehab and requested to speak with her mother's nurse. A nurse, April, came on the line and had some difficulty hearing on the phone because as she answered she said, "hello, hello?" Mara answered and introduced herself.

"I am just calling to get an update on my mom. How is she doing?"

"Well, I wasn't told that there were any issues overnight and she hasn't had any complaints so far during my shift."

April sounded quite busy and distracted. She spoke quickly and did not encourage conversation. It sounded like she was not expecting to have to respond to questions about residents.
"Okay great. Thank you. Will you please let her know that I called?"

April replied, "Yes. Okay. Bye."

***

It was busy at work, but when she saw there was a call with a Virginia area code on her cell phone, Mara left her desk to take the call. It was a young lady, Melanie, who introduced herself as a physical therapy student at the Alexandria rehab.

"I met your mom and she told me that I could call you to ask some questions about her. Was your mom able to do anything for herself before she got sick?"

"Yes. She was independent."

"Did she use any assistive devices like a cane, walker, wheelchair?"

"No."

"Who does she live with?"

"Her son lives with her."

"Are there any steps to get into her house?"

"There are about three steps outside."

"What about inside? Any steps?"

"There are about twelve steps to her bed-room."

"How does she get to appointments?"

"I take her or Metro Access."

"What is the plan for her when she's ready for discharge?"

"She will return to her home or to my home. The plan is to get her as close as possible to her baseline."

"Alright. Those are all the questions that I have. Thank you so much for taking my call. Have a good day! Bye."

"Thanks. Bye."

***

Mara got off work, at her work site in Germantown, Maryland. She got in her car and sat for a few minutes. *Okay. Let me see my mother.*

The rehabilitation center was in a different direction and was, for Mara, at a shorter distance from both home and work than the long-term acute care hospital. However, there was more traffic to contend with.

As Mara entered her mother's room, she noticed that she was watching television. Denise was looking at the news and the story was about political changes. Denise shook her head to whatever she had heard on the news. She clearly had an opinion. She was happy to see Mara. She smiled. Mara leaned over her mother's bed, and they embraced. They spoke about each other's day. Mara mostly wanted to hear about her mother's day.

Denise told her, "There were a lot of people in here today. Staff, I mean. Apart from the nurses and nursing assistants, a physical therapist, occupational therapist, and speech therapist. A student too but I do not remember if she is with the physical or occupational therapist. They said they were just introducing themselves and the student stayed a bit longer to ask some questions."

This was real progress. *Wow. I cannot believe mummy is able to tell me all of this.*

Mara told her mother, "I spoke with Melanie earlier today. She is a physical therapy student."

"Okay, she's nice," Denise said.

"Anything else happened today?" Mara asked.

"No. Just these crazy people on tv. I am tired of being away from home. What is going on with you? Anything new?"

"Nothing is new. Just work as usual."

Denise looked at her daughter from head to toe, "Okay missy, I need you to go buy some new clothes." She smiled.

"Mummy, what's wrong with my clothes?"

"Mara." She shook her head and gave what her daughter interpreted as a disapproving look.

"Okay, mummy. Let's exercise a little."

She really sounds like she is back! Even criticizing what I am wearing! She is tired of seeing me wearing the same outfits.

Mara moved the sheet to the foot of the bed. She pointed to her mother's right leg. Denise was sitting upright with the head of the bed at about a forty-five-degree angle. She began to lift the right leg off the bed. She counted one, two, three. She paused. She looked up at Mara. She continued—four, five, six. She paused again. She continued until she got to ten.

"Now the left, mummy."

Denise lifted the left leg. She struggled. She could not get it high off the bed. Without saying anything, Mara leaned over the bed and put her hand underneath her mother's left heel. She lifted the left foot. Denise continued to try to lift her leg. This time it seemed easier for her. They counted— one, two, three…all the way to ten. Mara moved closer to her mother's left arm. It was resting on a pillow.

"Lift this arm." Denise lifted her arm a few inches off the pillow.

"Good! We just have to keep practicing mummy."

"Yes," Denise replied.

Mara looked at the fingers. They were still curled inward, touching the palm of her hand. She tried to open the fist, but Denise squeezed her eyes. She put her right hand to her forehead and bit down on her lips.

"I am so sorry, mummy. I am trying to prevent these fingers from staying like this. I will stop."

She rubbed her mother's hand. She looked around the room. Where is the splint? She wondered. A nurse walked into the room.

"Hello. Do you know what happened to the splint that my mom should be wearing?"

"A splint?" The evening nurse responded. "I didn't get report about a splint."

"Mummy did you have it on today?"

"No. I don't think so."

Mara looked in the top drawer. She found it inside of the chest of drawers and placed it on top of the chest of drawers so that it would be visible to the staff and so that they would adhere to the schedule.

"There's a schedule for the splint." She told the nurse. "She needs to wear it during the daytime, and it should be removed at 5pm."

The nurse replied, "Okay. You need to speak with the therapists about that."

Why would she need to speak with the therapists? Was it routine for families to contact every discipline separately? This seemed to be a different approach. Was there no communication between nurses and therapists for the nurse to feel as though she could speak to the therapy department on her patient's behalf?

Mara was concerned about the splint. She knew that whenever the splint was not applied to Denise's left hand for even a day, that is, the schedule that was initially created, it became more difficult to apply it the next time because it was painful for her. Her fingers were contracted and attempts to straighten them caused significant pain. She massaged her mother's fingers and applied lotion to her dry skin. She looked at the time on her phone. It was 7:56pm.

"They are going to kick me out soon. Let us pray. Thank you, Lord, for giving us another day to spend together. Please protect mummy and guide those caring for her. This we ask in Jesus' name. Amen."

She leaned over the bed and hugged her mother. Denise kissed her on her cheek, "get home safe." Mara smiled and nodded.

***

From work the next day, Mara called the rehabilitation center to check on her mother. Nurse Vera came on the line and introduced herself as Denise's nurse.

"Your mom is okay. From the report that I received, she had a good night and so far, no problems during my shift."

It was mid-morning and Mara was pleased to hear the report from Vera and hopeful that the entire day would go well for her mother.

At the end of her workday, she shut down her computer, picked up her handbag and walked down the hallway. She met Judy, one of the nurses, in the hallway, "Lucky you. You are leaving already" Judy said.

Mara laughed. "It is the end of my shift, lady. I have places to go. Have a goodnight."

Judy smiled, "goodnight, Mara."

She got in the elevator on the fifth floor. The doors opened on the first floor, and she walked out into the parking lot. There was a little breeze. Mara got into her car. She thought to herself, "Let me find some music so I won't think of this horrible traffic."

Interstate 270 south in Germantown is usually not bad at this time of the day but Interstates 495 and 395 are horrible. She put a Beres Hammond CD on and smiled. Traffic was heavy but Beres was playing so things were not too bad. She sang along.

"I see love from a distance, coming but slowly. I know it's gonna last forever. I feel us coming closer, closer, and closer. It's the time we get together."

She arrived at the Alexandria facility. The lobby was empty. She took the elevator down to her mother's unit on the lower level. There were a few nurses sitting at the nursing station.

"Hello" she said. One of them responded, "hello." She walked into her mother's room. Denise smiled when she saw her. She walked over to the bed and gave her mother a hug. Soon after she arrived, Denise's friend Jenice was standing at the door. Denise saw her. She opened her mouth as though surprised to see Jenice. Denise smiled. Jenice walked over to the bed, and they embraced. Denise had not been aware that her friend had planned to visit her. She continued to smile. She stared at Jenice.

It was now July 2017, eight months since she had been away from her house. They spoke about all sorts of things.

Suddenly, Denise said, "There was a man in here last night. He was dressed in a red suit and was jumping on my bed. The man just kept jumping all over the bed. I told him; careful you fall on me."

They laughed at Denise's description of the man in the red suit. "You were probably dreaming," Both Mara and Jenice told her.

She did not dispute that it could have been a dream. She said, "But it seemed very real." Mara thought:

I wonder if they are giving her medications that would cause her to have this type of dream. She is hallucinating, or it was a dream. The transfers from one facility to another was too much for her brain. She has been through so much.

Mara made a mental note to follow-up to see if this dream reoccurred or if anything similar happened with her mother. The "man in the red suit" did not come back. Mara only heard about it again later when Denise told other visitors about that experience. Each time that she described the man in the red suit, she laughed uncontrollably. This always triggered a coughing spell. The little loud ventilator alarmed.

Chapter 31

Addressing more issues

It was five in the evening. Mara's workday ended. She shut down her computer and walked to the elevator. I really hope traffic is not bad, she thought to herself. She walked out of the hospital. Wow, it is still bright and sunny out here. She got in her car and put a soca CD in. *I need to get gas*, she said to herself. She drove to the gas station about three traffic lights away. She filled up the tank. *Okay mummy, I am on my way.* As usual now that Denise was in Virginia, she was driving from Germantown, Maryland to Alexandria, Virginia. Tapping her fingers on the steering wheel to the beat of the music, she thought, traffic is heavy, but it is moving.

She parked in the open parking lot at the facility. A lot of cars here. As she picked up her phone to put it in her bag, she looked at the time. It was ten after six. There were a few people in the lobby. She waited at the elevator. It was slow. She entered her mother's room. Denise was sitting on a wheelchair next to the bed. *Good. She is out of the bed. But why is she in such a small wheelchair? I wonder why they did not put a pillow behind her back.*

"Hi mummy." She walked over and hugged her mother.

Denise was sitting with her right arm on the armrest. The television was on the news channel. She was leaning forward with her right hand supporting her head. She looked up. She did not smile. Her face showed that she was uncomfortable.

"Hi dearie. Girl, I am in so much pain. I have been sitting in this chair for an hour."

"Oh no. Did you tell your nurse?" Mara placed her hand on her mother's shoulder.

"I pressed the button, but I haven't seen anybody."

About two minutes later, a young man entered the room. He was dark complexioned, of African descent. He was broad-shouldered and about five feet, four inches tall. He wore navy blue scrubs. He looked directly at Mara. He smiled. "Hello. I am Harry. I will be the nurse this evening."

"Hi. I am Mara, her daughter."

Harry looked down at Denise. He smiled. "Mama. How do you feel?"

Denise looked up at him; she sighed, "I need some pain medicine. I am having back pain."

Harry looked concerned, "Okay. I will be back with your pain medicine."

He walked at a normal pace out of the room. Mara watched him. *"Oh oh. He just went into the room next door! Maybe he is just going in there quickly,"* she thought.

She continued to look at the doorway. After several minutes, Harry walked out of the other room. He walked down the hallway, in the direction of the nursing station. *Okay. He should be back soon with her pain medicine.* Denise stared down at the floor. She sighed.

"Oh, my back." She clenched the armrest of the wheelchair.

They waited. Forty-five minutes went by. Mara kept pacing and returning to her mother's side. She watched the doorway. She walked to the door and looked out, peering right along the corridor. Eventually, in the room, she pressed the call bell. Several minutes passed. An older dark complexioned African man, Bada, he said his name was, walked into the room. He was the nursing assistant. He was about Mara's height, five feet, one inch. He had a questioning look on his face.

"Yes? How can I help you?"

"My mom is waiting for pain medication."

Bada opened both palms facing upward, "The nurse was here, did you tell him?"

"That was quite a while ago and my mother is having severe pain."

He had a serious expression. He held his chin with his right hand, "I will tell the nurse."

Another ten minutes passed. There was still no Harry with the pain medication. Mara walked out of her mother's room. She paused and looked down the hallway. The nursing station was at the end of the long hallway. Harry was sitting at the nursing station with Julia, another nurse. As Mara approached the two nurses, they kept their heads down, looking at a schedule.

"Can we help you?" Julia looked up and asked.

"Harry, we're still waiting for pain medication."

"Yes, I am coming."

Mara paused, looked at him, opened her mouth to say something, then turned and walked back to her mother's room feeling helpless. At 7:20pm, a full hour since Mara had heard Denise complain about pain and ask him for medication, Harry walked into the room with Tramadol. He had a blank expression.

"Mama, I have your pain medicine." Could this be cultural? This refusal to even acknowledge that something was out of the ordinary. But no; she had seen poorly administered care in other facilities and an uncaring attitude did not seem to have a culture. She was thinking this now because both the incompetence and the blank stare that accompanied it annoyed her. Ordinarily she would understand. She was in no mood to be the understanding one. And calling her "Mama" might be cultural but now it particularly annoyed her. *Don't call her Mama if you're not treating her like a mother should be treated.* "Harry, she has been waiting for an hour." Mara said. He made no response. He simply turned and left the room.

Bada walked into the room a few minutes later. He had the hoyer lift. He looked at Denise, "I'm going to put you back in the bed." She nodded. He attached her to the hoyer lift, lifted her off the chair and put her in the bed. He wheeled the machine closer to the door, turned and said, "goodnight." Mara responded, "goodnight."

Denise closed her eyes and dozed off to sleep. Mara looked at her phone. It was 7:55pm. She kissed her mother and left, expecting that after such an ordeal she would be asleep for a long time. How, she wondered, could one feel comfortable leaving relatives in a facility like this?

On July 12, 2017, the following day, Mara called the unit. The unit manager, Edna, answered. Mara said, "I had planned to give you a call because I need to speak with you."

Edna replied, "Oh, okay."

"I was visiting my mom yesterday evening and she was having excruciating back pain. She told Harry that she needed pain medication because her back was hurting her. It took one hour for Harry to return with pain medicine. I eventually had to find him, and he was sitting at the nursing station. In the meantime, my mom was crying in pain."

Edna told Mara, "I am sorry. I will talk to Harry."

"Okay. Thank you. Can I speak with my mom's nurse?"

"Yes. It is Viola. Hold on."

Viola came on the line. She told Mara, "Your mother was complaining of chest pain, and I gave her tramadol. The physical and occupational therapists were both in to see her, but I do not know how she did with them."

Her mother's therapy, Mara knew, was confined to her room as she was on isolation. It was hard for her to imagine how much therapy could be done in that small room. It was more conducive to performing exercises in the bed. Was that the extent of the therapy?

At approximately 3:45pm on the same day, Mara received a call from nurse Soni.

"Your mom was found unresponsive at 1:30pm but she's okay now."

Mara was worried. 1:30? Why hadn't they called to say something? It was good to know that her mother had regained consciousness, but what had happened?

"How long did she remain unresponsive?" she asked.

Soni responded, "I don't know."

The nurse did not have any more information. Perhaps everyone was busy trying to determine what had caused the unresponsiveness. Perhaps they were also busy documenting the occurrence. She wondered if they had considered transferring her mother to the hospital.

"Okay. Thanks for letting me know. If anything, out of the norm occurs again I would like to be notified sooner," Mara said.

"I am sorry. She is okay." Soni replied. "Yes, we will call sooner if anything else happens."

That evening, Mara saw her mother and she was stable, no complaints. The visit with her mother was as usual. They spoke about the day's events. Denise had no recollection of being awakened after the unresponsive incident. Mara allowed her mother to rest, instead of exercising. They prayed together. The voice on the intercom came on at 8pm.

"Attention all visitors. Visiting hours have ended. Please use the side doors on the first floor to exit the building. Have a good evening."

Mara kissed her mother, "good night mummy."

"Good night. Get home safe."

Chapter 32

Transfer to Alexandria hospital

On July 13, 2017, early in the afternoon of the next day, Mara received a phone call from the social worker, Jolly, at the Alexandria rehab.

"Your mom was complaining of chest pain and so she was transferred out to the Alexandria hospital."

Mara held her breath for a few seconds. She put her hand up to her chest. "Thanks for letting me know."

She was glad they transferred her to the hospital and left work early because of her mother's emergency. She rushed to her car. She turned on the GPS and put in the address of the hospital to which her mother had been transferred. Traffic was light and she got to the hospital in under forty minutes. She met her mother in the emergency room at the hospital. There was a bedside table next to the stretcher with crackers and juice. Denise was eating, drinking, and talking! Mara paused. Her diet at the rehab was via the gastrostomy-jejunostomy (GJ) tube in her abdomen and she was not allowed to have anything by mouth. Mara opened her eyes wide. She stared at her mother, thinking that she must really have improved a lot. Or did they just not know? It was several months since her mother was able to eat or drink anything by mouth. Had they checked, she wondered. What was happening? She talked to Karen, the emergency room nurse.

"She has not been allowed to have anything by mouth at the rehab. Did her diet change?"

Karen wore dark blue scrubs. Her badge said RN. She was a Caucasian lady, in her mid-thirties. She wore her hair in a ponytail just past her shoulder. She was surprised.

"I was not told that she was not allowed to have anything by mouth."

Mara looked at her mother. *She has quite an appetite, but I wonder if she told them that she was not eating by mouth at the facility. Perhaps she did not understand or even know to say something. She probably thought that her diet had changed.* Karen told Mara, "To be honest I am not impressed with that rehab facility. We always get patients from there and many of them have pressure ulcers. I am glad to see that your mom does not have any pressure ulcers."

Mara was alarmed. Pressure ulcers? "My mom just transferred to the facility for rehab and weaning from the vent, but I'll make sure I continue to remain involved in her care."

As a nurse herself, Mara was worried. She watched her mother continue to eat. She thought to herself, I hope this does not set her back. It is worrisome about the amount of communication there is between facilities. Mummy could aspirate. She should be evaluated by speech therapy to make sure that it is safe before they allow her to eat by mouth. How do they know that it is safe for her to eat? We do not want food to go into her lungs.

Her mother's friend, Audrea, walked into the room. Denise was being admitted. They waited for what seemed like an eternity for a bed to become available on the step-down unit. While they waited, one of the emergency room physicians walked in. He smiled. He wore a long white lab coat. He stood next to the stretcher on Denise's left side. Next to the physician was a young man who held a laptop in his hand. He wore a plaid shirt and a pair of beige pants. Mara looked at both men. *That must be the scribe*, she thought, as she looked at the younger man. The physician walked a little closer to Denise.

"Hi there! You just had a major heart attack!" he told her.

His voice was loud. He looked concerned. Denise stared at him. She looked over at Mara and Audrea. She opened her eyes wide. Her mouth opened. Her chest started to rise quickly.

Audrea said, "It is okay Denise. Try to relax."

Mara said, "You are okay Mummy. You're okay." She rubbed her mother's arm. She looked over at the physician. Her eyebrows furrowed. The scribe said something quietly to the physician. He looked at the laptop that the scribe was holding.

"Oh!" he said. He cleared his throat. He put both hands on the stretcher and leaned over. He dropped his voice and said, "I am sorry. I am mistaken. That was someone else's chart. But your troponin level is elevated. Okay, well you take care." He nodded, smiled, and walked out of the room.

Mara sighed. She stared at the doorway. What just happened? She wondered. Did he even verify her identity? I do not remember him saying his name. Are doctors not expected to introduce themselves to the patients? Do they normally check to make sure that they are talking to the right patient? I really hope that my mother does not actually have a heart attack now. She rubbed her mother's hand, while she stood next to the stretcher. She looked down at her mother. Her chest was still moving fast.

Karen walked into the room, "Okay. So, we have a bed for you upstairs. You will be going up shortly."

A few minutes later, Karen walked back into the room with a young Caucasian woman. She was also wearing the RN badge. She smiled. She was in her early twenties. Her hair was pulled back in a ponytail. She wore the same color scrubs as Karen. She did not say anything.

A young African male wearing gray scrubs came in with a portable monitor.

"Hi" he said as he looked at Denise. She responded, "Hi." He walked to the head of the stretcher. He put the monitor on the stretcher and transferred the connecting wires from the monitor on the wall, near the head of the stretcher to the portable one. It was only then that Mara looked at the setup and realized that her mother was on full ventilator support. They wheeled her and all the equipment out of the room. Mara and Audrea followed them on to the elevator. They got to the second floor, turned left, and they saw the nursing station on the right after the turn. They got to the first room, and they wheeled her into the room. One of the nurses said to Mara and Audrea, "Give us a few minutes."

They pulled the curtain. Mara and Audrea waited in the hallway outside of the room. Mara looked to her right, and she saw her friend Sharon, walking down the long hallway toward her. Sharon was wearing a long loose-fitting black blouse, a pair of blue jeans and black sandals. She was smiling. In her hand was a brown plastic bag. She got closer. She hugged Mara and hugged their auntie, Audrea.

"I brought you dinner," she said to Mara and handed her the plastic bag.

"Oh. Thank you." Mara smiled and took the bag. These attentions from friends were a huge part of the support system for Mara.

***

Denise was placed in a semi-private room, but she was the only patient because she was on isolation. The nurse who had asked them to wait came to the door. She was of Middle Eastern descent. She had a long black ponytail and a bright smile. She said, "You guys can come in." They put on the isolation gowns and walked into the room. Denise was still breathing fast but her breathing had slowed down from when she was in the emergency room. She was sitting at about a forty-five-degree angle in the bed. She smiled when she saw them.

The nurse said, "My name is Shonda. I will be your nurse tonight. This is my number, and this is the phone number to the unit." She pointed to the phone numbers written on the white board on the wall at the front of the room. "Visiting hours are from 7am to 9pm." It was a little past 9:30pm, but they were allowed to visit without anyone making it an uncomfortable visit for them.

Mara met the physician who was rounding. Dr. Raina was a South Asian middle-aged woman. She stood at the doorway and gestured to Mara to meet her outside of the room. Dr. Raina asked Mara questions about her mother.

"How long has she been living at the rehabilitation facility?"

"She does not live there," Mara answered. "She recently transferred there for short-term rehabilitation. I noticed that she was eating regular food by mouth in the emergency room, but she was not at the facility."

With raised eyebrows, Dr. Raina said, "I am concerned about her aspirating and so I would place her back on the tube feeding and nothing by mouth."

Mara also provided her mother's medical history to the physician. Audrea, Sharon, and Mara visited for a little while and then wished Denise a good night. Mara told her mother, "Mummy I'll see you tomorrow."

Denise had a sad look on her face, but she tried to smile and said, "good night."

***

On the following morning about 10am, Mara called her mother's nurse to check on her status. The nurse told her that it had been an almost sleepless night for Denise.

"Your mom did not sleep much during the night. So, she is still asleep."

According to nurse Katelyn, her vital signs were stable while they were talking but her blood pressure and heart rate had been elevated during the night. Her laboratory results were normal. Mara told the nurse, "Please let her know that I called and that I'll see her this evening."

***

On July 14, 2017, after her workday ended, Mara drove to the Alexandria hospital. Her mother's expression said that she was happy to see Mara. She was receiving her tube feeding and was on the ventilator. Mara remained optimistic that her mother would be free of the tube feeding and the ventilator one day.

"You are doing well. You are getting there mummy. Just keep working toward returning home." Denise responded with a nod. Mara stayed past visiting hours. She met the night shift staff. She assisted the nursing assistant to turn her mother in the bed and made sure that she was comfortable before she left. Mara was almost at home when she received a phone call from the Alexandria hospital. It was the night nurse.

"The cardiologist wants to talk to you," she told Mara.

Dr. Maynor came on the phone and sounded quite upset or concerned. "Your mother has some type of behavior that I do not understand. She is banging on the bedrail, and it seems as though she wants someone to stay in the room with her, but the nurses are quite busy. We will need you to return to the hospital."

The description of the 'behavior' was familiar. Had personnel at the facilities talked to one another? She knew that it happened. Was this the anxiety track?

He said, "She is agitated."

"Can you please put my mother on the phone?" Mara asked Dr. Maynor.

Denise came on the line, "Mara, everybody here is so nice but my stomach is really hurting."

Mara listened carefully. But she is speaking clearly, she thought. There is no difficulty in understanding what mummy just said. She opened her mouth in surprise. The fact that I can understand what she is saying, means that he can as well. He is standing right next to her. He could ask her what is wrong.

"Mummy just rub your stomach. Can I talk to the doctor again?"

Mara told Dr. Maynor, "My mother is having pain. Please give her some pain medication."

Mara wondered, "Did he even ask her what was bothering her before he had the nurse call me?"

"I would order something for pain and something else for agitation."

Why were the facilities so eager to medicate for anxiety? Were they afraid of people? She did not understand what was happening. She was almost at home. She was exhausted and just wanted to get home, shower, and go to bed. She figured that her mother would be okay after being medicated for pain and 'agitation.' More than likely she would fall asleep. Mara got to her house. She checked her mail. She had received a letter from the Baltimore facility. What can this be about now, she wondered. Mummy is no longer at their facility.

The letter read:

July 13, 2017

Dear Ms. Mitchell,

Thank you for voicing your concerns with the Nursing Supervisor and Manager of Guest Relations regarding the experience your mother shared with you while she was a patient at Baltimore Long Term Acute Care Hospital. I appreciate you sharing as you did on her behalf. We welcome the feedback and take it seriously. The Nursing Supervisor met your mother, and the investigation was initiated. The Nurse Manager also met with your mother to get additional information.

Additionally, our team interviewed staff involved with your mother's care. I am sorry to hear the perception she described. I wanted to inform you the findings were unsubstantiated due to insufficient evidence.

I appreciate you bringing her concerns to our attention. I apologize for her described experience. If you have any additional questions, please feel free to contact met at 410-000-0000.

Sincerely,

VP, Patient Care Services/CNO

Although disappointing, the response was truly not surprising to Mara. She also realized that the letter suggested that she had reported her mother's complaint; however, her mother had made her own complaint and it was done while visitors were with her. She wondered whether she should point out that the complaint had not come from her. It was not unusual that there would be no admission by the facility to inappropriate behavior of any kind by a staff member to one of their patients. She would not have expected them to admit any wrongdoing, but a simple acknowledgement of their patient's feelings would have been the humane gesture, she thought. They could have apologized directly to Denise for her discomfort and reassured her that they were interested in her safety. The experience was an unpleasant one for Denise, not for anyone in administration or their family member or relative. At least it was no more than the way that she was held that made her feel uncomfortable. Mara was upset but pleased that that was all that her mother reported. She believed that her mother felt uncomfortable, which was the reason that she told her daughter and her two friends. I wish I could clone myself, she muttered. I cannot do everything, but I wish I could. As she thought about her mother's experiences, she remembered what her Auntie Myrna kept telling her when her mother was at the Baltimore facility: Mara, be gentle on yourself. You live a whole hour and more away from the hospital. You cannot be there all the time. Listen to your body, too, you know.

What the facility had done was ensure that Manuel was not assigned to Denise's care anymore. Unsubstantiated. What does that mean? What does it ever mean? Do they think my mother does not know anything? If she is uncomfortable, she is uncomfortable. Did they find out if anyone else is uncomfortable? Are they looking at him? How are these things best handled? Mara had told her mother to let her know if anything else occurred that made her feel uncomfortable. She never reported anything else. Mara continued to visit her mother daily. She always remained polite and professional with the staff. She asked questions when relevant and requested assistance for her mother when necessary.

She held the letter in her hand. She sighed. She looked up and said, "Lord, help us." She put the letter down on the kitchen counter. She had some chamomile tea. She went upstairs, took a shower, and started to get ready for bed. She decided that she should check on her mother's status at the Alexandria hospital one last time, before she went to sleep.

Denise's nurse Shonda told Mara, "I was just about to call you. Your mom has not calmed down. I have not been able to leave the room because your mom continues to bang on the siderail. So, we will need you to come back."

Mara did not know what to do. Come back? She was at the other end of the I-270, in Maryland. At the best of times, it was a long enough drive, but now, when she was so tired, it would be impossible. She picked up her handbag and started walking down her stairs. She puffed her cheeks and blew out some air. This is so ridiculous, she thought. At times like these, there should be someone else to help. She stepped out into her garage and got in her car. She looked at the time. It was 12:20am. At least traffic will not be a problem at this hour, she thought. She remembered how to get there but still turned-on Waze for the alerts. She put in a soca cd to help to stay awake. Soca was particularly useful these days. I-270 south was almost empty. It was the early hours of Saturday morning. There was some traffic on 495 and then 395 but the traffic was moving. She drove thirty-five miles back to Alexandria, Virginia from Germantown, Maryland. What could she do? She was dog tired. But how could she not go? She rubbed her temples with the tips of her fingers. She did not want her mother to be mistreated because she displayed a behavior that no one understood.

Why didn't they understand her behavior? What, she wondered, was so unusual?

On her arrival at the hospital, the security officer, a tall African man with broad shoulders told her, "You can't visit at this hour."

It was 1:06am. She explained, "I was asked to come to the hospital. My mom is Denise Mitchell. She is on the second floor. The nurse called me."

He called up to the unit and was told that Mara was permitted to visit. She took the escalator. She arrived on the unit. She walked quickly down the hallway and got to her mother's room. Her mother was asleep. She watched her, the gentle rise and fall of her breathing. She stood watching her. There were no nurses around. The light above the head of the bed was bright. I'm glad she's comfortable, but did I have to drive back here thirty five miles because the hospital doesn't really care? Shonda walked in.

"Let's let her know you're here."

"No. Let her sleep. That is not necessary."

"No, I think she should know."

She walked over to Denise, tapped her on her right shoulder and said, "Ms. Mitchell, your daughter is here." Denise opened her eyes, smiled, and went back to sleep.

"If that ever happens again, I will not return to the hospital for that purpose. This hospital must have a solution for when patients have pain and have not had any relief from the pain medication."

"I am so sorry, but I did not know what to do. I could not attend to my other patients. Your mom was given additional pain medication after the initial dose. You could sleep in the next bed."

Mara walked to the other bed in the room, sat down, slid the shoes off her feet, and lay on her side watching her mother. Then she just lay there and counted the hours. She looked at her phone occasionally as another hour went by. Her mother remained asleep. Mara could not sleep. Shonda walked in. Mara looked at the time on her phone—7am. Another young lady came in with her. She was African American with a very pleasant smile. She held a clipboard in her hand.

"This is Beverly. She will be the day nurse." Beverly waved and said, "good morning." Mara replied, "good morning." She looked over at her mother. She was still asleep. Mara smiled.

Mara stayed at the hospital until other visitors arrived. Her mother complained of abdominal pain again once the pain medication wore off. As Denise had mentioned, everyone there was nice but, to Mara, no one was interested in trying to determine the cause of the abdominal pain. She was getting ready to leave when Dr. Maynor walked in. She had spoken with him over the phone, the previous night. He was a Caucasian man, in his mid-fifties and stood about six feet tall. Mara recognized his voice. He said to her "Thanks for coming back to the hospital last night. You know, it was difficult for the nurse to attend to her other patients."

"I am sorry to hear but I really did not think that it was acceptable that I was asked to return. I came back because I am concerned about my mother. My house is not next door to the hospital."

He opened his hands with palms up. He looked down at Mara, "I am sorry, but I was at my wits' end. Where are you coming from?"

Her face was serious, "Germantown."

"Oh. A bit of a drive, huh?"

"Yes, it is."

He clasped his hands together. "The medication seemed to have helped. She calmed down after she got a second dose, the nurse told me."

Mara thought to herself, if every patient were to complain of pain and were not relieved with the ordered pain medication, there would be a family member in every room, every night.

They stood at the foot of the bed, facing Denise. She was looking at them. She had a blank expression. Mara continued talking to Dr. Maynor. "I don't know if you know my mom's medical history."

She paused and looked at him.

"I read some of it from her chart," he said, looking down at her.

Mara, thinking, *I do not know what is in the chart.* She took a few moments to explain her mother's medical history for what felt like the 100th time. But she had to explain in detail and bring up the new concern about the abdominal pain.

She realized that he was the cardiologist and not the attending. He was amenable to listening to Mara's comments and questions. He told her, "I will order a CT scan of her abdomen and a CT of the chest."

"Okay. Thank you," Mara said.

He looked down at Denise and smiled. He then turned to Mara and said, "Good talking to you." He walked out of the room.

A couple of days passed. Mara followed up with her mother's nurse, Monica. The CT scans were done. Monica told Mara that the physician would provide her with the results.

On July 19, 2017, both CT scans were negative. The tube feeding was suspended, and Denise's complaints of abdominal pain were not as severe. The pain became more tolerable for her. Mara wondered if the tube formula was the cause of the abdominal pain. The physician who was rounding was Dr. Tesfaye. She asked him if he would allow her mother to eat. He ordered a speech therapy's consult. The speech therapist performed an evaluation that included a swallow evaluation. Denise passed the swallow evaluation. She was placed on a mechanical soft diet by mouth. She tolerated the diet. The physician at the short-term rehab, Dr. Kulkarti, was also her attending at the hospital. Most of the patients who were transferred to the hospital from the rehab remained under his care. Since Dr. Tesfaye was the one rounding, Mara spoke with him about her mother's care. He suggested that the chest pain was a result of the chest compressions that Denise had received in the ambulance when she was transferred to Simion Hospital.

Later that day, Mara received a phone call from Dr. Kulkarti who was visiting other patients at the hospital and was following up on Denise's status.

He told Mara same as the covering physician said, that the chest pain was because of the chest compressions that Denise had received. Then, without apparent reason—at least, no reason that was apparent to her, he said, "Your mother may need to consider changing her code status to do not resuscitate." *Another one!*

He explained, "If she had to receive chest compressions in the future, she would experience chest pains." Mara listened. She looked at the phone. She said quietly, "My mother's code status will remain full code." The fact that her mother complained of chest pain was surely not reason for her code status to be changed to do not resuscitate. She would, however, appreciate relief from the pain. Mara wondered if he realized how ridiculous and insensitive his comments were. In his experience, it was an unusual occurrence for patients who have had chest compressions from CPR to complain of chest pain. Was he sure that that was the reason for the pain? Why were they all so quick to suggest a Do Not Resuscitate code?

Denise's stay at the hospital was extended but the reason was unclear to Mara. The physician on call told Mara that the chest pain was because of the chest compressions and the abdominal pain was related to the tube feeding. Although she did not enjoy the food, she was happy that she was allowed to eat. She started to make friends with the staff and knew their names and schedules. That was not unusual for her. She soon kept in her thoughts identifying details about people. She was seen by the physical and occupational therapists at the bedside. Any information that indicated progress on Denise's part had not been transferred along with her, or the staff at the long-term acute care hospital as well as those at Northern Metropolitan Hospital where she started to make some progress, were simply unwilling to acknowledge the information.

To avoid her mother being maintained at the same level by the facilities and repeating the same pattern with no progress, Mara knew that she had to communicate information that was important. She made sure that the therapists knew that her mother had sat in the chair for a couple of hours per day at the long-term acute care facility. There was no hoyer lift on the unit and it required some searching to obtain one from another unit. When the hoyer lift was brought to the unit, the staff told her that she would be transferred to the chair. The nurse and nursing assistant attached Denise to it and began the transfer. Denise started to panic and called out to the male Ethiopian nurse Yash. She called out, "Yash! Yash!"

She was fond of him. He reassured her "You are okay, Ms. Mitchell. You will be okay."

She kept her eyes on him and was placed in the chair. Mara sat next to her mother and updated her on events of the day. Before Mara left her mother, the nurse offered to transfer Denise back to the bed and Denise agreed. The nurse and nursing assistant prepared her for the transfer to the bed and she was calmer than she had been when she was transferred to the chair. Once she was settled in the bed, Mara said prayers at her mother's bedside. She waited for her to fall asleep and then sent out a text:

Hello everyone, mummy was transferred from Alexandria Rehab to Alexandria Hospital room 2523A. She has been complaining of chest pain and since the rehab is not equipped to handle that, they sent her to the hospital. She is stable. I am sorry for the late notice. Thanks for the continued prayers.

She wished the nurse a good night and headed home.

***

The next day, Mara made her routine trip to the hospital at the end of her workday. She reached her mother's room shortly after she had been transferred to the chair. She met her mother's friends Breana, Lori, and one of her friends Mikala at her mother's side. They encouraged Denise to eat and although it took some time, she ate a moderate portion of her meal. She enjoyed the company of her friends as she sat in the chair. They spoke about people, places and events that were familiar to her.

"You know, Denise, I hear that Daphne's daughter is getting married," Lori said.

Denise raised her eyebrows. She smiled. She said, "Oh, yes? That is nice. Who is she getting married to?"

Lori said, "A guy from St. Lucia. He seems nice. I have not really spoken to him."

The staff periodically checked on Denise, and she was content that she had her visitors at her side. The staff reminded them that Denise was only allowed thickened liquids. She tried to convince them that she was able to drink the liquids without the thickener, but they followed the staff's orders. Breana, Lori, and Mikala visited for about two hours and said their goodbyes to Denise. She seemed sad but understood that they had to go to their homes. After they left, Denise told Mara, "I must cook and invite everyone to come over."

Mara realized that her mother was a bit confused. She agreed and told her mother, "Yes, when you get well."

Denise gave her daughter a questioning look. Mara re-oriented her mother, "Mummy this is 2017. You are at Alexandria hospital. You're here because you were at the Alexandria rehab, and you were having chest pain."

Denise acknowledged with a nod and did not say anything else on the subject. They watched television for a little while. Mara called their family in Grenada via facetime and Denise spoke with her mother, sister, and brother. They were all smiling. Her sister Yvonne told her, "You are coming along well. Your face looks good."

Denise smiled. She said, "thank you." Her sister-in-law Lina said, "You are getting tired. Okay. Have a good night."

She nodded her head. They ended the call. Mara pressed the call bell as she thought that her mother would be more comfortable sleeping in the bed. One of the nurses responded promptly. She informed them that she would call other staff members to assist. Within minutes, Yash, a nursing assistant, Rita, and the nurse Carla returned. Yash explained to Denise, "We will put you back in the bed. Do not be scared okay. You will be okay."

They attached her to the hoyer lift. She kept looking at him. They transferred her to the bed. She smiled and said "thank you" to them. Mara continued to sit at her mother's side. Denise fell asleep and felt guilty about not being able to stay awake. She woke up a few times. She apologized to her daughter, "Sorry Mar. I keep falling asleep."

"You need to sleep. Go ahead, sleep."

Her mother did not take her suggestion. She was clearly trying to stay awake and keep Mara company. Mara realized that her mother would try to stay awake if she continued to sit there. She told her mother, "I am getting ready to go. You need to rest. Let us say a prayer."

Denise was on full ventilator support and her voice was audible. They said the Lord's prayer together.

"Okay Mummy. Have a good night."

Denise, as she was used to prior to being hospitalized, wanted to make sure that Mara had gotten home safely. She said to Mara, "call to let me know that you made it home safely."

"How? You remember you are in the hospital, right? You do not have a phone."

Denise was not to be outdone. She showed that she could problem-solve for her daughter. She said, "call my nurse and he could tell me."

They both smiled and Mara left. She knew that her mother would not sleep well if she did not call. When she got home, she called the night nurse who was in Denise's room at the time. He put her on speaker and Mara was able to say, "Mummy, I made it home okay. Sleep well."

Mara sent out group text messages as usual to update everyone and to continue to request prayers. Denise remained at the Alexandria hospital for a couple more days. Her electrolytes were abnormal, and she was administered potassium and magnesium to increase the levels. She continued to receive occupational therapy at her bedside. Mara continued to advocate to encourage the weaning process. The respiratory therapists were receptive to her input and worked diligently to advance Denise with the weaning. The physician who was rounding prepared Mara for the discharge to the rehab. There was not much else to do at the hospital. The chest pain was attributed to the chest compressions when she received CPR and the abdominal pain was a result of the tube feed formula, they believed.

Denise was to be transferred back to the rehab. Mara met her mother at the hospital and reminded her that she was returning to the rehab. Everyone was nice, as her mother said, but it was time to work toward returning to her home. It seemed like another stop to allow Denise to be cared for by a multidisciplinary team that made her feel as though they cared about her. Of course, nothing was perfect. There were a few exceptions.

Chapter 33

Transfer back to Alexandria rehab

On July 25, 2017, when Denise arrived back at the Alexandria rehab, Mara was asked by one of the nurses to wait in the dining room on the unit. It took several minutes again for the assessment to be completed. The assessment at the rehabilitation center was more thorough than it was at the hospital. That was odd because Mara recalled being told by more than one of the nurses at the hospital that they received many patients from the rehab with pressure ulcers. If that were true, that meant that the facility was more skilled in determining whether patients had any skin breakdown, than actually preventing them. When the assessment was completed, one of the nurses told Mara, "You can go in to see her now."

Mara got to her mother's side and Denise was hysterical. She was crying and wanted to go home. She told Mara, "They kidnapped me. We have to go now."

Denise started to try to get off the bed, as Mara tried to console her and explained to her, "Mummy they did not kidnap you. I will not allow anyone to kidnap you. You are back at the rehab. You cannot get out of the bed. You are not strong enough."

Mara realized that her mother was confused again. Denise had been transferred several times in a short amount of time, so she found it difficult to adjust. She insisted, "Mara we have to go now."

Mara realized that her efforts to convince her mother that she needed to stay there, were ineffective. She called her aunt Breana as she figured that her mother would listen to her friend. She explained to Aunt Breana, "Mummy wants to leave the rehab. She thinks that she was kidnapped, and she is trying to get out of the bed. I am trying to convince her that she needs to stay in the bed."

Breana spoke to Denise, "Denise, you cannot get out of the bed okay. You are not strong enough to support your weight. If you get out of the bed, you could fall, and you will hurt yourself. You may break your hip. That will just delay your recovery." As Breana told Denise some of the consequences that could occur if she got out of the bed, Denise nodded her head in agreement. It was not a facetime call. Mara interpreted the head nodding and told Breana that her mother agreed. As soon as they got off the phone, Denise started again, "Mara let us go."

She continued to cry. It took several minutes before Denise calmed down. She explained to Mara, "the nurses told me that I am not allowed to leave the bed. They were very harsh and loud."

Oh! So, their attitude triggered this behavior. That was very upsetting for Mara to hear but she simply embraced her mother and tried to reassure her that she would be okay. Mara explained to her mother, "they meant that you can't get out of the bed without assistance."

It was difficult for her to explain other people's intentions and behavior when they themselves did not make any effort to communicate effectively and with empathy. Oh, my goodness, she thought. The panic is starting again because she is back here. What did they tell her when the door was closed? How does one deal with the health system when things like this happen? No wonder it felt like a kidnapping! What was she to do? She reiterated what Aunt Breana told her. She begged her mother, "Mummy just do what the nurses tell you to do because every day is a day closer to you coming home."

Denise nodded. Mara stayed with her mother for a while longer. They watched television and shared a few laughs. Denise had a long day. She became sleepy but forced herself to stay awake. She tried to keep Mara at her bedside by asking about everyone whom she thought about. She started to make different complaints of discomfort such as wanting to change positions in the bed and wanting to use the bathroom. It seemed that whatever she thought about that would keep her daughter at her bedside longer, that was what she did. She was obviously afraid to be left alone with those who had the responsibility for her care. Mara encouraged her mother to go to sleep after they prayed. It took several minutes before she finally fell asleep. Mara sent out the text messages to update everyone and to request prayers.

Mara checked on her mother's status the following morning. At the Alexandria rehabilitation center, there was a lower level of confidence among the nursing staff, with a higher vocal tone than what she observed at the Alexandria hospital and at Simion hospital. Mara was used to looking at the trends in her mother's laboratory results and vital signs. She asked specific questions such as what the vital signs were and the vent settings. The nurse responded, "she's good, everything is good."

Mara could not understand why it was difficult to get responses to those specific questions. She asked the nurse, "Were there any changes to the ventilator?"

There was silence.

"Have they started weaning her from the ventilator?"

Again, the nurse was not able to provide an answer.
She told Mara, "You would need to speak with the director of respiratory services."

That seemed odd to Mara, that the nurse was not able to provide information about her patient's weaning and felt that she needed to defer to the director of the respiratory department. Mara was not familiar with the various roles at the rehab and accepted that it was routine for the director of respiratory services to be the one to provide her with updates. This was quite different from the attitude at the hospital Denise had just left. The hospitals make a difference, she thought. Why do they have these attitudes? This does not at all feel like a caring profession. Does it mean that they are less trained here? The nurse told Mara, "Mr. Carlton is the director of the respiratory department. He is right here. He can talk to you."

Mara said, "Thank you" but then she realized that the nurse had already handed the phone to Carlton.

Carlton said, "Hello. This is Carlton Hanes, director of respiratory. How can I help you?"

"Hi Carlton. My name is Mara. Denise Mitchell is my mother. I am checking on her status. I have been following my mom's progress closely and would like to know of any updates with the weaning from the ventilator."

"The weaning has not started yet. With it being so close to the weekend, I would feel more comfortable being here when her ventilator settings are changed."

Mara was slightly disappointed but also appreciated his concern and attentiveness. She was certain that there was a reason for that and a reason for him being the one to provide her with information. While her mother was at the Alexandria hospital, one of her mother's respiratory therapists had suggested that she should ask the physician at the rehab to change the current type of tracheostomy to a shiley, which was a different type of trach than what was in place. He had also suggested that she request that a medication called mucomyst be ordered for her mother's thick secretions. She did not understand why she should have to ask the physician to order anything. He was a pulmonologist, as well as her attending physician while she was a patient at the Alexandria hospital. He would know what her mother needed. A few days prior to speaking with Carlton, she left a message for him to convey her messages to the physician. They had not spoken about the message in the initial conversation, but Carlton had called Mara back to inform her that he would follow up with the physician.

Mara continued to call the Alexandria Rehab to get daily updates. She lived and worked too far away to just stop by whenever she wanted. Her schedule only allowed her to see her mother when she had completed her workday. The day shift at the rehab had ended by the time she arrived in the evenings and usually the response from the evening nurse was, "I don't know."

She arrived at the facility at about the same time every evening. The staff quickly figured out her schedule. That was not necessarily a good thing.

Pain medication

Strangely enough, there was a repeat of the incident with deprivation of pain medication. Harry had not been assigned to Denise in several days. Mara was at her mother's bedside and again, Denise complained of back pain. Mara encouraged her mother, "press the call bell."

After about fifteen minutes, Harry responded to the call bell. Denise told him, "Harry, my back is hurting. I need some pain medicine."
After Harry left the room and did not return for several minutes, Mara left her mother's room to find Harry. She could not find him, and no one knew where he was. Mara asked to see the charge nurse and that person was busy helping with an admission. The wait for the pain medication

lasted for almost an hour again. This was obviously done purposely. Could there be some justification for such inhumane behavior? Mara reported that incident to the unit manager again. Edna's response was, "Harry again. I spoke with him the first time. This time I will have to do more."

Mara was certain that performance was just that…a performance. Mara realized that if Harry's behavior was occurring in her presence, she did not want to imagine what occurred when she was not there. Was there a certain type of personality seeking employment at this skilled nursing facility?

She was angry now, but also afraid to show her anger because this was where her mother had to be housed for who knows how long. These facilities, she reflected, can have tremendous power because they are in demand.

The rehab was more accessible to Denise's work friends. Many of them lived in Virginia and Washington, D.C. They visited, so that was one positive. Denise was happy to see friends whom she had not seen in months. They updated her on the latest news from the office. Mara was happy that her mother was closer to everyone. She worried about her feeling lonely and depressed. The Baltimore facility was further away from her family and friends and although she had visitors, the visits were sporadic and consisted of the same group of friends. Mara knew that her mother's spirits would be lifted if she saw her family and friends often. She would also be more engaged, and the staff would... hopefully...have no reason to medicate her for depression.

***

One day, when she had just finished a report at work, Carlton called again. He informed her, "the tracheostomy would not be changed until your mom is more stable. The ventilator is set at SIMV, and this allows her to breathe in between the ventilator rate. Also, she got mucomyst today and that will help to thin out the mucus."

Mara realized that her mother had regressed with the weaning. She did not know if her mother's status with the weaning was as a result of the several transfers from one facility to another, or whether it was as a result of the therapists' own assessments to determine what she was able to tolerate or if it was due to inaccurate documentation that was sent to the facility, as well as, inaccurate record keeping at the facility. Carlton told Mara, "Feel free to call for updates. I will also call with occasional updates."

Mara did not want to become a nuisance. Her thought was that the director would be too busy to have time to provide her with updates. Carlton made himself available to all the patients. He was directly involved in patient care. Mara observed that about him when she visited her mother in the evenings after work, as she usually did. He stayed late at times. He checked on patients. He spent time with the patients, families, the respiratory therapists, and the nursing staff. At the facility, the patients were referred to as residents. Mara never subscribed to that and continued to refer to her mother as a patient. She did not want to suggest that that place would ever become her mother's new home. She would not become a "resident." But was that the conflict? Did it benefit them in some way to have patients and families thinking of the facility as a "residence?" Was that what it was intended to be? Did staff, knowing this, try to ensure that people became residents? Was this about the business?

Preventing pressure ulcers

Denise was comfortable speaking with Carlton. She discussed her care with him, and he got used to reading her lips. It was possible that he did not always understand. He did not appear to be one who would want to hurt her feelings, so if he did not understand her, she never knew. Denise did not realize that she was not always continent of urine. She was continent of stool. As far as she knew, she would let staff know when she needed to use the bathroom. The type of care that she received was not very consistent and as a result she was even more confused.

One day when Carlton and Mara were at the bedside, Denise asked Carlton, "Do you know this lady, Vanessa, who works at night?"

Carlton said, "Yes." Vanessa was one of the nursing assistants.

"Is she interested in women?"

Mara opened her mouth and her eyes wide. She was shocked and embarrassed at her mother's question and responded, "Mummy, Carlton cannot answer that."

At her baseline, she would not have asked questions along those lines. Carlton nodded in agreement with Mara's comment. Denise explained, "She shows too much interest in me. She is always saying that she is checking on me and even when I say no, she says that she must check to see if she needs to clean me. It is strange that no one else comes in here as often as she does at night."

Carlton asked Denise, "Did anything strange. happen?"

"No. She comes in here too much. The other people check on me at the beginning and at the end of their shifts sometimes."

Mara quietly thought, "*Oh. That makes sense. There's inconsistency in the type of care that she is receiving. It is confusing to her.*"

Mara was embarrassed. She said to her mother, "Mummy, Vanessa is doing what she is supposed to do. That is her job. She is not being inappropriate. She needs to make sure that you are clean and dry."

Denise shook her head. Carlton said, "I'll discuss this with Edna."

Within an hour, Edna, the unit manager was at Denise's bedside. Denise repeated the same story to Edna.

As they discussed the issue, Edna suggested, "how about we produce a schedule for Vanessa to check on you a little less frequent?"

Denise replied, "Yes. Okay."

Edna smiled and said, "Okay. Vanessa will check on you twice during the shift."

Denise did not seem pleased, as though twice may have been too many times but she smiled and said, "okay."

Mara looked at Edna and thought to herself, "*Well I suppose that is the reason for the many pressure ulcers if what the Alexandria Hospital nurses said is true. She needed to be educated about her situation but that did not occur in the conversation with Edna. Frequent checks were necessary since she was not always aware of when she needed to receive personal care.*"

Mara knew that meant that she had to check her mother's skin more thoroughly to ensure that there were no issues such as skin breakdown. If the comments by the nurses at the Alexandria hospital were true, allowing patients to lay in their wastes for hours overnight, which was the pattern at the rehab, would help to explain why many patients had pressure ulcers.

Confused

While at work, Mara made her usual call to the Alexandria facility to get an update on her mother's status. The nurse informed her, "Your mom was found sitting on the floor next to the bed!"

The nurse was speaking very loudly. She heard the tone of annoyance as the nurse informed her, "I told her to call for help and it looks like she was attempting to get up to go to the bathroom! She does not have any pain and she said she did not hit her head!"

Mara realized that the nurse did not realize or did not care whether that was a patient whose brain had been through significant trauma. Denise had periods of confusion. At times she did not remember that she was unable to ambulate by herself. She needed to be reoriented to her environment. The tone that the nurse used made

Mara worry. She hoped they did not yell at her mother or mistreat her in any way for not following instructions at the rehab. Mara informed the nurse, "You know she has suffered a few strokes and she does not always remember her limits. I will talk to my mom when I see her."

The nurse's response was simply "okay," to the comment that Mara would speak with her mother. Mara was uncertain as to whether the nurse grasped the concept of the effects that the strokes may have had on Denise. It was either ignorance or lack of care or concern. That was one of the reasons why Mara was not in a hurry to have her mother transfer to a skilled nursing facility. Skilled is the operative term here but skilled in what?

Denise needed more time in a safe and amicable environment to allow her to recover before transferring to a skilled nursing facility that provided a lower level of care. Unfortunately, the long-term acute care hospital from which she had been transferred was neither safe nor amicable.

Chapter 34

Awareness

On August 1, 2017, the social worker, Jolly, called Mara to say that they were scheduling a care plan meeting for August 9, 2017, at 4pm, a week later. Mara would have made plans to be present in person, but she worked in Montgomery County, Maryland and the rehab was in Alexandria, Virginia, thirty-five miles away. The driving would be too much.

"I'm sorry but I won't be able to leave work to attend." Jolly replied, "No problem. Would you be accessible by phone?"

"Yes."

Jolly said, "I will put a reminder in your mom's room. The meeting will be on August 9th at 4pm."

In preparation for the care plan meeting, Mara jotted down a few questions that she wanted to ask the team. Where is she with the weaning? How is she with therapy? Does she get out of bed to the chair? Is she on any narcotics? It was her first care plan meeting. She did not know what to expect. She was hopeful that the call would not be as previous phone conversations that she had with health care personnel. In the past, she found that they really wanted to give information, not to listen. It seemed more a monologue than a dialogue. She wanted to ask the question about the narcotics because her mother was extremely sensitive to narcotics and would sleep for extended periods whenever the nurses medicated her with narcotics. The continuous drowsy state prevented her from participating in her own care.

At the end of her workday, Mara visited her mother. Denise was awake and was watching television. She was happy to see her daughter. They spoke about the events of the day. Mara said to her mother, "I heard that you were sitting on the floor. What happened?"

Denise told her daughter, "I do not remember. I just remember the nurse being upset with me. She told you?" She was not expecting that the nurse would tell Mara about her being on the floor. Mara wondered whether her mother felt that way because of how upset the nurse was or whether the report made her feel like a child being reported on. She did not want to focus too much on the nurse's reaction but hoped that the nurse's behavior was professional. She remembered the tone that the nurse used on the phone earlier in the day as she reported that Denise was found sitting on the floor. She sounded to Mara as though she was shouting. Mara reminded her mother, "Mummy I do not want you to get hurt. You are not strong enough to walk. Whenever you need anything press the call bell for help." Denise nodded. They performed a few exercises. Again, Mara applied lotion to her mother's skin. The evening nurse entered the room and told Denise, "I have your medications."

Mara introduced herself, "Hi. I'm Mara her daughter. What is she getting?" The nurse seemed surprised by the question and stared at Mara for a moment but named the medications as she gave them. Was the question unusual? She knew that it was her mother's right as well as hers to know what medications she was about to receive. Perhaps so few people asked that when someone did, it was beginning to seem to the nurses like an imposition. Mara wanted to avoid another calamity with her mother's medications. Are we getting the same type of training in nursing school? Is the nursing care supposed to be different in the rehab setting than in the hospital? Mara stayed at her mother's bedside until visiting hours ended. They said prayers together and Mara left the facility.

Care plan meeting

On the day of the care plan meeting, Mara received a phone call from Jolly. Others present at the meeting were Edna, the nurse manager on the unit, Dr. Kulkarti, the attending physician and pulmonologist, Amber, one of the physical therapists and Veronica, the dietician. Jolly explained, "Everyone will present as it pertains to their discipline and Mara you can ask each person questions if you have any."

Edna presented first. "She is getting Vancomycin until August 22nd. The podiatrist came on August 8th and trimmed her nails. She does not have any pressure ulcers but there is some redness at the bottom of her heels."

Mara asked, "Is she receiving any narcotics?" Edna replied, "I'll have to get back to you. I do not know if she is on any narcotics."

Mara then said, "She had been out of the bed to the chair at the Baltimore facility. Is she getting out of the bed to the chair?"

Edna responded, "That I do not know. You will have to ask the therapists because they would be the ones working with her with that."

Next, Dr. Kulkarti presented. "She is doing well with the weaning. I plan to take her off the ventilator completely tomorrow," he said. There was no need to ask the physician a question, Mara thought, because he already said that her mother was doing well with the weaning.

Amber presented, "the therapists are working on bed mobility training with Denise. She requires maximum assistance with transfers." At that point, Denise was on isolation, so she was confined to her room and that was where she received therapy. She responded to Mara's question about being out of bed, "we are focusing on bed mobility only. She is not being transferred to the chair."

Lastly, Veronica spoke about Denise's nutrition. She said, "she lost a couple of pounds. She would benefit from more nutrition. Perhaps some liquid supplements and a snack every afternoon."

The meeting did not last much longer. They wished Mara a good afternoon and the call ended. Although she was not pleased with some of the answers she received to her questions, Mara acknowledged that they had been addressed.

Chapter 35

Keeping in touch

On August 9, 2017, after the care plan meeting, Mara contacted the insurance case manager, Toni. She did not want to have any surprises regarding her mother's stay at the rehab. She also did not want the case manager to forget about Denise. She left a voicemail message for Toni.

"Hi Toni. This is Mara. Denise Mitchell's daughter. I wanted to be in contact and to find out if she has any more days available for rehab. Please give me a call when you get a chance."

Toni called the next day. "Your mom continues to meet criteria to receive care at the rehab. She does have more days remaining." Mara was glad to hear that her mom could continue to receive care at the facility, but she forgot to ask about the exact number of days remaining for rehab.

Denise did not tolerate being off the ventilator completely from the day after the care plan meeting, as Dr. Kulkarti had planned. She continued to propel toward being free of the ventilator but was not there yet. Every day she tolerated being with the trach collar for more hours than the previous day. Denise's many visitors encouraged her to relax during the weaning process. She had a history of panicking whenever she realized that she was not on the ventilator. She had been on the ventilator for such a long time that her body had grown accustomed to it. Carlton was very patient with Denise and her weaning. A few of the respiratory therapists were patient as well. Mara was grateful because she knew that there were other patients at the facility who needed attention.

She had to admit to herself when she thought about it that those other patients were not her mother. She could not get involved and advocate for them, but it was her responsibility to advocate for and ask questions about her mother. After starting the entire weaning process all over again, Denise had surpassed the level that she had accomplished at the long-term acute care hospital. When she visited her mother, she reminded her, "Mummy remember your goal. You want to be discharged to home without a tracheostomy and without oxygen."

Mara knew that it was not an impossible task. Her mother had gotten too far to become complacent and to allow anyone to place limits on her. It had taken a long time to reach that point but Mara knew that everyone had a role to play to succeed with the weaning process and for her mother to be safely out of Alexandria rehab. On the family's and friends' end, prayers, support, involvement in care and advocacy, were needed. The multidisciplinary team at the rehabilitation center, she expected to be competent in their roles, compassionate, patient, and professional. Thinking of her own training, Mara felt as if she were required to teach. She felt that it was a challenge to encourage some of the health care personnel to function appropriately in their roles. There were many occasions when it seemed obvious that they had no interest in working toward positive outcomes. The lack of interest was evidenced by the slow responses to Denise's or her visitors' requests for assistance, poor pain management and infrequent rounding by the nurses and respiratory therapists. All of this made her think about her own job and the way she thought about those committed to her mother's care.

***

On September 6, 2017, while at work, Mara received a phone call from one of the physical therapists, Jaimie, and an occupational therapist,

Ellen. *Oh good!* She thought when she heard who was calling. *I've left at least two messages in their department for them to call me. I want to know about mummy's therapy schedule.*

The therapists told Mara, "We have been trying to reach you for about two weeks."

Mara thought their statement was outrageous. Of course, they had not been trying to reach her for two weeks. She was at the facility every day!

"I have not missed any calls from Alexandria rehab." Mara replied. "What number have you been calling?"

"The same one we're calling now."

She knew that she had never missed a call from the rehab. She told them, "I am interested in knowing the schedule for my mom's therapy. I can attend sometime."

Jaimie described Denise's therapy session. She told Mara, "Your mom requires one person's assistance in and out of bed to the wheelchair. We attempted to use a sliding board for the transfers, but we were not successful. She tolerated sitting up for about thirty minutes."

As Mara listened, she knew that her mother had sat up for longer than thirty minutes before she transferred from the Baltimore facility. Jaimie continued, "Her oxygen saturation dropped significantly lower than 90% so we had to stop working with her. We do not think that she can tolerate this level of care. We can reassess in a couple of weeks."

A couple of weeks! Mara asked, "What was the exact oxygen saturation when it dropped?"

Perhaps surprised by Mara's question, Jaimie responded, "I don't have the exact figure with me."

Ellen the occupational therapist then said, "I would recommend that a washcloth could be used in your mom's hand to help to keep her fingers from continuing to curl inward. We want her to be more stable before we work with her again."

Mara inquired from the therapists again, about the incident in which her mother's oxygen saturation dropped, "I am really concerned about that day when her oxygen saturation dropped. There must be something that caused that. Do you know if she was seen by respiratory?"

The therapist told her, "Well that is all we know. You will have to talk to her nurse."

It seemed to Mara that they had provided all the information that they had planned to provide. Mara was concerned that her mother needed to be suctioned by staff or that the inner cannula of the tracheostomy needed to be cleaned. She was curious to know whether her mother had been seen by respiratory therapy before the session and what the circumstances were that caused her mother's oxygen saturation to drop. She was not given an opportunity to provide her opinion. The therapists had already decided that Denise should be bedbound, or wheelchair bound a couple of weeks. That was too much time to allow to pass without active therapy. They had not suggested a day or two for her mother to miss therapy sessions. Their suggestion was to take a break for a couple of weeks. The progress that her mother had made would be forgotten by her own body, and she would regress.

Later that afternoon, there was another care plan meeting scheduled. The individuals who attended were Jolly the social worker, Veronica the dietician, Dr. Kulkarti, Carlton the director of respiratory therapy, Jackson the assistant nurse manager and Mara via phone. Carlton discussed the tracheostomy tube and said, "the trach tube was changed to one without a cuff. If she does not tolerate the plugging from the trach, she may need to be seen by ENT (Ear, Nose and Throat specialist)."

There was no one from the physical therapy department present at the meeting. Jolly presented on behalf of the physical therapists. Earlier in the day when Mara spoke with the therapists, she was told that they would reassess her mother in a couple of weeks; however, at the care plan meeting, Jolly reported, "per the therapists, she has plateaued." Mara was surprised to hear that. It meant that her mother had reached her maximum potential and that she had done as well as she would do with therapy. They had not told her that. And what were the factors motivating their decision? She only became aware of the therapists' evaluation at the care plan meeting. Mara was amazed. It seemed to her that everyone was being dishonest. Was it because she knew a bit about that area of work and could tell when they were being dishonest? She began to wonder about this. Was this something to do with long-term care or acute care generally? Why first at the long-term acute care facility and now at the Alexandria facility? Was it a general attitude that there was no room for people who needed so much care? Was this how all these facilities functioned? She wondered if those levels of disinterest were requirements for employment at those facilities. Mara reflected on her conversation with the therapists and wondered what had prevented them from revealing their evaluation of her mother to her. She was concerned that their absence from the care plan meeting might have had something to do with the information that she had received from the social worker was different from what they had given her. Mara wondered if they realized the impact that their behavior would have on her mother's future. Mara was extremely disappointed. No one at the meeting said that they would advocate to have the therapists continue to work with Denise. What about Dr. Kulkarti? In her estimation, he had never openly demonstrated leadership in her mother's care. He sometimes provided a brief explanation or plan for changes with the weaning process.

"I am not a physical therapist, but I will come there and perform therapy with my mother," Mara informed them.

"But that's why we're here," Carlton responded.

Mara thought to herself, he was right. She realized that her 'to do list' had extended. She decided to contact the facility's administrator, hoping that someone at the Alexandria rehab had compassion and would put it to effective use.

Mara wrote a letter detailing her mother's medical history and everything that led up to that point. The most critical part she had to convey to the therapist was what could happen if she does not get regular therapy. She stated:

My worry with her not having therapy for weeks is that she will decline. Our plan is not for her to be a bedbound or wheelchair-bound patient. It appears as though that's where we're heading. I'm not sure how much improvement is expected if she is not actively participating in therapy.

It is unfortunate that now that she is free of infection and has improved significantly with weaning off the vent, the plan is to deny her therapy and seemingly allow her to decline. Once the providers give up on their patients who are fighting for good quality life, this lack of hope can be felt by the patients and families and as a result the patients give up as well.

I am confident that we can work together in addressing these concerns; with the hope that my mother will resume therapy soon. Thanks again for your efforts in trying to ensure that my mother gets excellent care at Alexandria Rehab.

Mara decided to write the letter because she felt as though it was a more effective mode of communication. There were many important aspects of her mother's care that she needed to address, and she did not want to omit any of it. She applied the same concept from her nursing knowledge, that if it was not documented, it was not done. She felt as though she was drowning in responsibilities that no one else would have been able to assist with, so to stay afloat she needed to communicate in writing to ensure that everything was addressed with veracity.

In addition to the letter, Mara realized that she would need to take on an even more active role in her mother's recovery. She spoke with the therapists at her workplace about her mother's situation. They did not understand the facility's rationale in deciding to suspend her mother's therapy sessions. They provided her with a crash course in therapy. She learned how to apply the gait belt and how to assist her mother with transferring from a sitting to a standing position and vice versa.

Chapter 36

Therapy

Mara continued to visit her mother at the Alexandria rehab. She explained to her, "Mummy, the therapists are no longer working with you but the two of us will do therapy daily."

Denise raised her eyebrows with apparent surprise but did not say anything. Mara brought her mother's wheeled walker from home. Denise had owned that walker since 2010 when she was discharged from the acute rehabilitation hospital, after the first aortic dissection.

Their initial sessions involved changing positions from sitting at the edge of the bed to standing on the side of the bed. Mara's friend Ania provided a standard walker, one without wheels, nonskid socks and a gait belt. The gait belt was used for the transfers. It was challenging at first but what they all wanted was to see improvement. After a couple of days, Denise felt comfortable enough to try to transfer from the bed to the chair with support from Mara. She was becoming stronger. She still needed assistance but less than she had needed a few weeks before. Mara told the nurses she would like her mother to sit in the chair daily. The staff used the hoyer lift when they transferred Denise from the bed to the chair and vice versa. Mara wondered why. She asked Jane, one of the nurses about the transfers. Jane told her that they used the hoyer lift so the staff would not feel too much of the strain. According to their physical therapists, Denise required one person's assistance to transfer in and out of bed; however, Mara thought that all of this was more about the facility than about her mother. If she required only one person, why was the hoyer lift being used? Wasn't their whole approach counteracting her own efforts and making her mother, who, she felt, could manage some of her own weight, less inclined to try? Both she and her aunt Breana requested a more comfortable chair for Denise to sit. Initially, the staff claimed that there were no chairs available; Aunt Breana, who knew the job and the system, insisted that the nurses provide a more comfortable chair. Mara arrived at the rehab one evening and noticed a new chair at her mother's bedside. She smiled. In her mind, she thought, *okay so they finally gave her a chair that would not cause strain or pressure on her back and buttocks.*

Now, Denise's family started to think that the rehab wasn't too interested in improvement for the patients. They thought there was something odd about the whole situation, as if it had already been decided that Denise was going to be a long-term care resident. Why would facilities not encourage patients to return home with families if that were their goal? Or could it be that was not their goal?

Denise was very motivated but the management and staff at the skilled nursing facility had grown accustomed to patients becoming dependent on them. It explained the surprise by the staff at the Alexandria hospital who had expected to see Denise with significant skin breakdown. Many of the patients who transferred to the hospital from the nursing facility, as Mara was told, did not have intact skin. Those patients were usually bedbound and dependent on staff. Denise had for quite some time now moved beyond that point. That was her appearance when she was at the Northern Metropolitan Hospital and the staff there expected her to remain that way.

In fact, Mara was beginning to guess, the expectation was that she would pass away in a few days, as would have happened if Mara had allowed for her to be taken off the ventilator. Mara knew that without her continuous involvement her mother would not have been able to participate in therapy with her. As she told the team at the care plan meeting, she would be there to provide therapy. She was a registered nurse, not a physical or occupational therapist, but she was now seriously considering getting some training as a therapist to take care of her mother. The little she was managing to do showed that her mother was able to work with her in the sessions. So of course, she thought, those who were formally trained as physical and occupational therapists should be able to help her mother to attain much more. It seemed, though, that was not to be.

***

On September 12, 2017, Mara got a response to the letter she had sent to the facility's administrator.

Mara,

I apologize for my tardy response. We have shared this information with the team yesterday (we were both out of the office on Wednesday and were not able to address your concerns). If our team has not reached out to you yet, they will be shortly.

Thank you for sharing your concerns and we look to bring resolution to them in the very near future.

The next correspondence that Mara had with the facility was on the same day after she received the administrator's letter. She received a phone call from the social worker, Jolly. The call was to inform Mara that a care plan meeting would be held in a few days. The participants at the care plan meeting were Jolly, Edna, Dr. Kulkarti, Carlton, Cindy, the director of physical and occupational therapy and Iesha the review nurse. Jolly led the meeting. Edna, the unit manager reported, "Ms. Mitchell sits up for a little less than two hours per day. She gets very anxious. Maybe she needs to be seen by the psychiatrist. That may help. What do you think?"

Mara knew that the question was being asked of her. "I have no objections to my mom being seen by a psychiatrist." Mara said. "I am concerned though about the anxiety I keep hearing about. I really do not appreciate the staff provoking anxiety that would result in her needing to see a psychiatrist. It seems as though she is being given sufficient medications for about three individuals. I would rather my mother not being on any additional medication that would hinder her ability to focus and to be able to participate in her care." There was silence. Then Carlton spoke. He said, "I am concerned about the desaturation event and so I placed Ms. Mitchell on continuous pulse oximetry monitoring. I scheduled an appointment for her to be seen by an ENT because she is still having difficulty tolerating the weaning from the tracheostomy."

Denise was at the point where they tried plugging the trach and she was expected to breathe through her nostrils; however, each attempt made, she failed as she gasped for air and her oxygen level dropped.

Carlton continued, "We attempted to change the type of trach to see if that would help but she could not tolerate the change." He finished by saying, "I would accompany her to the ENT's appointment." Mara was grateful.

Cindy, the director of physical and occupational therapy, suggested, "She needs to do some deep breathing exercises. The therapy department would re-screen her next week."

Mara was surprised by the contribution to the conversation from the therapy department. Next, Iesha presented.

"Ms. Mitchell's authorization from the insurance company has ended. I sent clinical documentation to the insurance case manager to request an extension of her time here at the rehab."
Mara was incredibly surprised. She had not called the insurance case manager in a few days, and this was both surprising and upsetting. She had no response to Iesha's comments. She would verify this information with the insurance company. This business of getting care seemed like a major battle.

"Mara, do you have any questions?" Jolly asked. Blindsided by all the information, Mara answered, "No, I don't have any."

"Well, we will wait for a response from the insurance. Your mom will be private pay if they do not give an extension. We will end here if there are no more questions. Oh, is your mother's code status still the same?"

Mara took a deep breath, waited a moment. "Yes, she is still full code…" Was it okay for facilities to appear to be covertly suggesting to family members that they let their relatives die? That is what it felt like.

"Okay have a good evening," Jolly said, before ending the call.

After the meeting ended, Mara immediately placed a phone call to Toni, the insurance case manager, to obtain more information and to request additional time for her mother to be allowed to have care at the nursing facility. The call went to voicemail. Mara left a message requesting a return call. A few hours later, Toni called.

"I reviewed the notes from the therapists. They stated that your mom requires total care and that she is appropriate for long term care."

Mara was more upset to hear this from Toni. She remembered Cindy's comment that the therapists would re-screen her mother the following week. Now, she was hearing that her mother should transition to long term care, which would mean that despite what she had been told, such re-screening was unlikely. Knowing how the system worked, Mara realized that if Toni had been given information that her mother was doing physical therapy, the decision could be different.

"I have been performing therapy with my mother at the facility. We have been working on transfers from the bed to the chair and back to the bed."

"Well, I don't have any documentation that supports that," Toni responded. "Talk to the staff and ask them to document what your mom is doing with you."

"Okay. I will. She is very motivated, and I cannot believe that they are saying that she should be a long term care resident, when she is making progress. Okay. Thanks Toni. I will."

They ended the call. Mara decided that she would speak with the nurses at the facility to request that they document what they observed her mother do with her. So, they had stopped therapy and although they knew that her daughter was doing it, with satisfactory results, they refused to acknowledge or document this. Since they were the authorized health care facility, this meant that their report had more weight with the insurance company.

Mara's understanding of the process was that if her mother converted to long term care and lived at the facility, she would no longer receive skilled services such as physical and occupational therapy. This was now about finance and payments. The facility was arranging to be paid to take care of a patient to whom they would not have to provide skilled services.

Mara left a voicemail message for the insurance case manager to inquire about coverage for the ENT appointment that Carlton had scheduled as well as transportation for her mother. She had not received a return call but knew that her mother needed to have that appointment, so she planned to make the payment for transportation. Carlton called her.

"We tried again with the plugging of the trach, but I am sorry your mom did not pass. I confirmed the ENT's appointment and scheduled the transportation. I gave the company your phone number so someone will call you for the payment." Mara responded, "Thank you Carlton."

The ENT's appointment occurred two days after the care plan meeting. There was no response from the insurance case manager; therefore, Mara proceeded with the payment for transportation and hoped that the ENT's visit would be covered by the insurance. The result of the examination was that there was some swelling and possible granulation tissue within Denise's airway that prevented her from tolerating the weaning from the tracheostomy. The specialist suggested that the swelling be decreased with medication and if not resolved in a month, Denise may need to go to the operating room. The plan for the operating room was to remove excess tissue that was preventing her from tolerating the tracheostomy from being plugged and for her to breathe through her nostrils. Mara wanted to avoid the operating room.

***

On September 20, 2017, another care plan meeting was held. A few of the same participants were present. Mara, as usual, was at work, so she participated over the phone. Carlton reported, "We changed the tracheostomy to a different kind and a smaller size." He stated, "I would try to plug the trach tomorrow."

Mara continued to listen. Veronica, the dietician presented. "Ms. Mitchell lost a few pounds."

Mara knew that her mother did not like the food at the facility and so she was not surprised by the weight loss. With permission from the nursing staff, Denise's family and friends brought food that she enjoyed as she was allowed soft foods. Veronica was aware of that and continued, "So I encourage the family to continue to bring food as long as it is soft foods."

Jackson, the assistant nurse manager, presented the laboratory results and said that her kidney function remained normal. After he provided the exact figures, he concluded, "All of her lab results are normal, including her white blood cell count."

Edna, the unit manager suggested, "Perhaps your mom can be brought out to sit in front of the nursing station to wait for you and then the two of you could have your dinner together in the dining room."

This suggestion was because of the staff's continued complaints that Denise wanted someone to be with her all the time. In addition to that complaint, Edna informed, "And she had another unwitnessed fall. The staff found her sitting on the floor near her bed."

Mara recalled being told about that incident by one of the nurses and she had spoken with her mother about it. Denise's explanation was, "I pressed the call bell and was waiting for a long time, but no one came. I was just trying to reach my eyeglasses and the table moved and the next thing I knew, I was on the floor."

Mara was relieved to know that her mother's bed was at the lowest level. It was so low that she would squat to be at eye level with her mother. At the meeting, Edna continued, "Whenever your mom sits in the chair in the room, she would ask to return to bed soon after. I think it would be better for her to come and sit in front of the nursing station until you come. What do you think?" Mara responded, "I think that's a good idea." Edna further commented, "I think that being away from the room, there would be less temptation for her to want to return to the bed."

Chapter 37

Oxygen saturation

    September 21, 2017 was a Thursday afternoon. Mara walked out of her workplace in Germantown. She got into her car at 5:15pm. She sat for a moment and massaged her temples. She put on a Duane Stephenson cd. She thought about her mother. She, too, enjoyed Duane Stephenson's music. She turned on Waze, again depending on the app to help guide her to the facility. She started to drive. There was not much traffic on Interstate 270 south. She drove down 270 and got to 495. The traffic was heavier there. The music was good. She focused on it and the drive went by more quickly. She arrived at 6pm. The lobby was empty. She took the elevator down to the lower level. Her mother was sitting in a wheelchair in front of the nursing station with her oxygen tank as she received oxygen via the tracheostomy. Denise smiled when she saw her daughter walking toward her. The nursing assistant wheeled Denise into the dining room and Mara carried her mother's dinner that was sitting on a tray on the ledge at the nursing station. Mara had also brought her own dinner from home. As they ate their meals, Denise seemed short of breath. Mara had seen a pulse oximetry machine in the hallway nearby on the way into the dining room, so she took it and checked her mother's oxygen level. She realized that it was in the mid-eighties. An acceptable level was 90% and above. She saw Ty, one of the respiratory therapists, sitting in the room next to the dining room. She waved at him through the glass doors and gestured for him to come out. He stood. He was an Ethiopian man. He stood about five feet ten inches tall. He was average build. She asked him to check her mother as she did not know why her oxygen level was so low.

He looked at her mother, asked "Are you okay?" Denise nodded yes. He then told Mara, "It is more important to see how the patient is doing rather than to look at the numbers."

Mara furrowed her eyebrows. But didn't the numbers *mean* something? Didn't they provide an alert that something might be amiss? He walked away. Mara was surprised that he was content with the low oxygen saturation and Denise's nod.

Denise's nurse Julia came by and looked at the pulse oximetry. She appeared concerned.

With raised eyebrows, she asked, "Ms. Mitchell, are you okay?" Again, Denise nodded but this time also mouthed the word "yes" and appeared to be short of breath. Julia left the room and returned with two respiratory therapists, one of whom was Ty, the therapist who had already spoken to Denise and Mara. The second therapist looked at the oxygen tank and turned it on.

Mara looked from one to the other and said to the therapists and nurse, "Please tell me what just happened."

The other respiratory therapist chuckled. She looked at Ty. She looked back at Mara. She appeared ashamed.

"You know what happened." Julia replied.

Mara knew but she wanted to hear them acknowledge it. Her mother had been sitting outside of her room for two hours with the oxygen tank turned off. No one had noticed. That explained the low oxygen reading. Since all three were together, she had better say something. "Now I am thinking that when she worked with the physical therapists and her oxygen saturation dropped, this is probably what happened. The tank was probably off." Mara looked at them and was not chuckling. Nothing about what just happened was funny.

There was no response to her comment. Mara also blamed herself. Why hadn't she realized that was the problem? Had she forgotten that she had to check the basics, even if this was not her workplace? To the workers at the nursing facility, her mother was not a priority, but to her she was. She should be more careful. After the oxygen tank was turned on, a few minutes passed, and Denise's shortness of breath improved. Fifteen minutes later, she was more relaxed. The two remained in the dining room until after they finished eating and then they returned to the room. The incident was alarming. These were the caregivers! This was where her mother lived now. She had to depend on the workers!

The wheelchair was not comfortable for Denise to sit in for extended periods. Mara helped her back to the bed. They spoke about their day and watched television until visiting hours ended. They said prayers. Mara sent out the usual messages, updating family and friends, and wished her mother a good night. She drove home with troubled thoughts. She put on a cd but could not focus on the music.

***

Denise was in good spirits whenever she had visitors. It was difficult to know what it was truly like for her earlier in the day when her family and friends were at work, and she did not have any visitors. She did not want Mara to worry about her and so Mara could not always depend on her mother being open about everything that bothered her. Mara was only able to visit earlier in the day on the days that she was off from work. Typically, she would have two weekdays off and on those days, she was able to spend more time with her mother. Denise had some regular visitors and she looked forward to their visits. Her friend Simon visited her every Saturday evening. She enjoyed his company. Hope was also a regular visitor. She prayed with Denise and gave her words of encouragement. Her friend, Andrina always made her laugh. Her sister Simone traveled from Grenada and Denise was happy to see her. Mart and Judlyn visited with their husbands and Denise was pleased. She said she could not wait to get out of the facility so that she could invite them to visit at home. She always felt better after she had visitors. Those who were unable to visit, both local and afar, sent their regards and Denise was just as excited to hear about everyone.

Her friend Mena brought an abundance of food. They ate together in the dining room along with Lori, Simon, Breana, and Mara. They had an indoor picnic as they talked and laughed about good times. Denise was overjoyed.

***

On September 23, 2017, Mara arrived on the unit and saw her mother sitting in front of the nursing station as usual. Standing next to her was a young man whom Mara did not recognize. Her mother was crying. Mara moved quickly toward her. There was another person standing closer to the nursing station. Mara had not noticed her at first. Now, she saw that it was her mother's friend. The young man she had seen on entering was Claudine's brother, whom she had brought along with her. Mara smiled to herself as she realized that her mother's tears were tears of joy. She laughed, too, because she realized she had been ready to ask the young man to step away from her mother. Denise had not seen these friends in a long time, and she was clearly happy. They went to the dining room together so that Denise could have her dinner. As they sat there and kept her company, Denise's neighbor in Gaithersburg, Frame, also visited and she was even more pleased. It was a good evening for her but a bit overwhelming because she was not able to sit up in the wheelchair for much longer. She had gotten tired and was ready to return to her room.

On September 24, 2017, just a few days after the incident in which Denise's oxygen tank was found to be off, Mara followed the nursing assistant with her mother into the dining room, as she had been doing since the plan was initially made for her mother to sit outside of her room. She brought the pulse oximetry machine that the staff left in the hallway along with them. She ensured that the oxygen tank was turned on. By this point, Mara felt that she was not simply being allowed the opportunity to visit her mother, she was a staff member. Although she would of course never resent having to do anything for her mother, there were days that she felt it would have been nice if she could just visit and enjoy her mother's company. She was constantly on lookout because she had little confidence in the care provided at the facility. She reasoned on those tiring days; she had a full-time job. She needed to ensure that she could perform there as expected. She was always tired after work and after a long drive. As they sat to have dinner, she observed her mother become short of breath again. She checked the oxygen level, and it was in the low eighties. She had already checked to ensure that the tank was turned on. What she failed to do was check the quantity of oxygen. She looked at the dial on the oxygen tank and realized that it was empty. This could not be happening! What was the problem at the facility? How often did things like this happen? Mara alerted one of the nursing assistants who was standing in the hallway, "Can you please tell the respiratory therapist that we need another oxygen tank. This one is empty."

The assistant responded, "I'll get a tank." A respiratory therapist came along with the nursing assistant. The nursing assistant exchanged the tank. They did not seem to think there was need for an explanation. She wondered again: how often did things like this happen?

On September 25, 2017, the Monday following the second incident, Mara called the director of respiratory therapy to inform him about what she observed with her mother's oxygen saturation. She told him, "While I was visiting my mom during this past week, her oxygen saturation dropped to the 80's. We were sitting in the dining room, and I asked Ty to look at her because her oxygen saturation was dropping. He asked her if she was okay, and she nodded yes, and he was okay with that. When the other therapist approached, she simply turned on the tank that had been off for hours. Then this past weekend, similar situation but this time the tank was empty." Carlton sounded very alarmed at what Mara told him. He responded "What? I would investigate these episodes as there was no documentation of either occurrence."

Mara was disappointed that the director of respiratory services was unaware of what she thought were significant incidents. No documentation. They simply did not write it up. No written report, so these things had not happened. So, performance at the facility could not be reviewed because reviewers did not have a real picture to work with! She noticed that updates she received from the nurses always indicated that her mother was stable, despite any distress that she was experiencing. One thing they regularly reported was anxiety, she noted, but they did not think it necessary to document something like that. If it had happened to her mother on two occasions, how often had it happened to other patients? What was the result? Had other cases been discovered and not documented, or not discovered at all until it was too late? Who would know?

What could she do? What choices did she and her mother have? What about families who did not have the knowledge to realize the problems with the oxygen tanks? And with other things. What about families unfamiliar with the hospital setting and, for example, with how an oxygen tank should work? Two respiratory therapists and a nurse knew of the first incident; none of them documented the first incident. In the second incident, the respiratory therapist who accompanied the nursing assistant to replace the oxygen tank with a full tank, also did not document the episode. Mara knew that she was only able to address the issues that she observed. If this was what she observed when she was there, what was the state of things when she was not there? It was frightening to think what all this implied about skilled nursing care and care for the elderly or extremely ill.

Chapter 38

Motivation

On September 27, 2017, Mara had not received an update from the therapy department since they had conducted their re-screen. She placed a phone call to the department and left a message for the therapist to provide her with an update on her mother's status. A couple of hours after having left the message, she received a phone call from Kim, one of the physical therapists. Kim explained that she worked with Denise on changing positions from sitting to standing. Listening to this, Mara knew she had also worked with her mother, practicing changing positions. Kim said that Denise marched in place and that she was motivated during the session. She had not been Denise's regular therapist. Mara was thankful for the update and realized, from some of the details given in the report, that Kim was not familiar with Denise's history at the facility. None of the therapists had mentioned before that Denise was motivated. They had reported that she was suitable for long term care. The previous therapist said that she could not tolerate that level of care at the skilled nursing facility. "Motivated." this therapist said. That was a good report.

Mara knew that her mother had the potential to recover. Denise was a fighter and was very motivated to get well. She wanted to return to her home or to live with Mara. Mara was open to her mother living with her. She thought about it now and tried to begin to make plans. She might have to figure out another arrangement. There were too many steps inside of her house and the design was not suitable for a first-floor set-up for her mother. They talked about it. Denise asked Mara if she would consider purchasing a different type of house that was appropriate, in which they could both have separate living quarters and privacy. That is an idea, Mara thought. Imagine! The suggestion had come from her mother! Mara realized that her mother was becoming more alert. She was able to consider issues and problem-solve to some extent. Importantly, she was showing interest in planning for the future. She acknowledged that she would need assistance when she was discharged but she also believed that she would be independent once more.

Moved by her mother's ability to look ahead and plan a future, and herself motivated by the support of others, Mara felt that prayers from those who cared about her, along with her determination, had allowed her mother to recover up to that point.

Together, she and Denise started to look online at houses. Denise assigned Mara to look for the home buyers' magazines, telling her where she should look for them—outside of the grocery stores or at newspaper stands. Mara was unable to find any of those magazines, so they continued to look online. It was an exciting project for both. It gave Denise something to look forward to.

Mara spoke to her mother about the possibility of going next to an acute rehabilitation facility as she had done in the past. An acute rehabilitation facility provides a higher level of care than at the Alexandria Rehab, which is a skilled nursing facility or sub-acute rehab. Denise was agreeable to that idea. She wanted to go to the same rehab in Washington, D.C. because, seven years ago, when she was transferred there, she thought they were excellent.

Mara also spoke with the insurance case manager who informed her that she would provide authorization for her mother to be transferred to the acute rehab, if she met criteria. Mara saw no reason for her mother to not meet criteria. She asked the social worker at the facility to send clinical information to two acute rehab facilities, one in Washington, D.C. and one in Rockville, Maryland. With the help of one of her coworkers, she got the contact information for a manager at the acute rehabilitation hospital in D.C. She informed the manager that she was interested in having her mother transfer to that rehab. There was some interest in the D.C. rehab accepting Denise, but they were reluctant to accept her because they were concerned about the tracheostomy and the fact that she had issues with it such as mucus plugs a few times. Mara did not understand their rationale because they had the resources to manage those issues, especially being connected to a tertiary care hospital across the street.

She also spoke with the liaison for the acute rehab in Rockville, who visited Denise at the Alexandria rehab. The liaison conducted her assessment and deemed Denise appropriate for her facility. She accepted her. That was great news because, as Mara was aware, the acute rehabilitation facilities had strict criteria for acceptance, and they believed that they were able to manage Denise's care. The problem was that although the therapists at the Alexandria rehab were verbally reporting to Mara that her mother was motivated and making progress, that was, after their hiatus from her care, their documentation did not support this conclusion. If only they were able to imagine themselves or their loved ones in Denise's or Mara's situation, would their behavior have been the same? Mara asked herself the question but had no answer for it. In January 2017, at the Northern Metropolitan Hospital, Mara had been told by Dr. Miles that her mother would remain in a vegetative state on the ventilator for the rest of her life and that was certainly not now the case. Denise was off the ventilator and breathing via the tracheostomy tube. Mara knew that her mother deserved a fighting chance. If you just leave it to some of these medical practitioners, they do not allow you to have that.

When she spoke again to Toni, the insurance case manager, she was told that they were documenting that Denise was appropriate for long term care. Mara pleaded, "Please give her the chance to go to the Rockville rehab. They have accepted her."

"I am sorry Mara. I could only provide authorization to the acute rehab based on the documentation from the Alexandria facility."

Mara was afraid that without therapy services, her mother would become less mobile. Mara then asked Toni, "Well, would the insurance send someone to the Alexandria rehab to conduct their own assessment?"

Toni responded, "No the insurance does not send anyone to the facility. The insurance relies on the facility to send information to support the services that the patients need to have covered."

Mara continued, "Toni, I don't understand this. My mother is not bedbound as you are being led to believe. She walks with me every evening in the dining room at the facility. We walk the entire perimeter of the dining room. She uses her walker, while I push a wheelchair behind her in case she needs to sit. I also push the oxygen tank. She tolerates more every day. She gets tired but we have the wheelchair with us."

"But we do not have any of that information. Can you please talk to the staff and ask them to document all of this?"

Mara was frustrated. Why wouldn't they document things that happened?

"They see us in the dining room every evening. My mom's nurses come in the dining room and give her medications there in the dining room. They tell her she is doing so well. It does not make any sense that they are not documenting it. I have asked more than one nurse to document our walks."

Mara felt that she had to let someone know that at this—and other facilities, a lot depended on what the facility decided was in its best interest. The patient was not the center of things. Agency lay with the facility, not with the patient and patient advocates.

Chapter 39

Denial of services

October 4, 2017, it was time for another care plan meeting. This time, Mara was able to attend in person as she was scheduled to be off from her job that day. They met in the dining room on the unit at Alexandria Rehabilitation facility. Present were Jolly, Dr. Kulkarti, Carlton, Edna, Jackson, Cindy, and Mara. They were all familiar with Mara. They waited a few minutes for Cindy to arrive before the meeting started. The nursing team Edna and Jackson presented, "Ms. Mitchell's labs are all stable." The team was aware that Mara was interested in having her mother transfer to an acute rehab as Mara had asked for documentation to be sent to the acute rehabilitation facilities and one of the liaisons came on site to assess Denise.

As Cindy sat down, Dr. Kulkarti asked her, "What is the possibility of Ms. Mitchell being able to tolerate acute rehab?"

Cindy seemed to Mara to be noticeably confident with her response when she said, "I do not think that Ms. Mitchell could tolerate three hours of therapy but may be able to do so in a few months." Mara was furious about Cindy's response. Mara understood acute rehab to be three hours of therapy per day, not three consecutive hours. Her mother had been to acute rehab in the past and had breaks between the disciplines of physical, occupational and speech therapies.

"The expectation is not for my mom to tolerate three hours of continuous therapy," Mara explained.

There was no response to her comment. She felt as though Cindy ignored her. Mara was there to hear the team's input on her mother's case, but she felt as though no matter how different their opinions were from hers; she would continue to advocate for her mother. She tried hard to dismiss her opinions about Cindy who appeared to not be interested in what she Mara had to say. Mara was not shy when she advocated for her mother. She resigned to the thought that there was no point in arguing with Cindy because she was allowed to have her opinion, no matter how ridiculous it seemed to Mara and how unfortunate it was for Denise. There were other issues that were related to her mother's care that needed to be addressed.

"I am concerned that my mother continues to complain about back pain daily." Mara said to Dr. Kulkarti. "I really do not want anything to be missed and for there to be any surprises with her health. It was complaints of back pain that caused her to go to the emergency room almost a year ago. I just want to ensure that a third aortic dissection is not on the way."

Cindy immediately responded as she furrowed her eyebrows and looked at Mara, "When does she complain of back pain? It is not documented."

Mara was awaiting a response from the physician to whom she had directed her concern. She continued to look directly at the physician and responded, "I don't know what is or is not documented, but I do know that my mother has been receiving pain medication every day for back pain."

Mara was becoming increasingly frustrated as she seemed forced to explain every comment she made. To her, the conversation was between herself and Cindy, and this was not her intention. Mara turned again to the physician, hoping that he would participate in this conversation, but he merely said, "I'll look into it."

The two nurse managers quickly started to look at their laptops and then simultaneously responded quietly, "Yes she has been getting pain medication." The nurse manager's and assistant nurse manager's low-keyed responses made Mara wonder what the nurses were documenting. She continued to think of other comments that she had intended to make to the physician. The tracheostomy had been in place for several months and the color of the secretions were a bit of a concern to her. She said to Dr. Kulkarti, "I think that my mother's secretions from the tracheostomy should be cultured. I do not like how the secretions look."

He was the pulmonologist. Mara was not comfortable with making those suggestions to the physician as she expected him to know what was needed, however, it seemed to her as though his visits to her mother were just that, visits. She was uncertain of whether he examined her. Once again Dr. Kulkarti responded, "I'll look into it." No one had anything else to add. The meeting ended.

After the meeting ended, Mara approached her mother's nurse Julia, and said, "Is it my imagination or has my mother been complaining of back pain? The director of PT said that it was not documented."

"I don't know what she's talking about," The nurse responded. Julia then opened the medication administration record on the computer and showed Mara where her mother received tramadol for back pain every day. *So, were they agreeing that the records show she had complained of back pain?*

Mara spent the rest of the evening visiting her mother. They went to the dining room where Denise walked the perimeter of the room, while Mara pushed the wheelchair and oxygen tank behind her mother. Denise was motivated.

Denise had been transferred from the acute care hospital to the long-term acute care hospital and then the sub-acute or skilled nursing facility. There started to be mention of her transitioning to long term care, in other words, nursing home resident while she was at the long-term acute care facility in Baltimore. That was when Mara became aware of the facility's plan for her mother; however, the idea, she felt could have been initiated at the Northern Metropolitan Hospital. She imagined that it must have been very unsettling for the Alexandria facility to hear from her that their plans were different from hers. It was likely that they were promised a patient who was being transferred to them for short-term rehab with the intention to transition to long term care. Being familiar with the role of transitioning patients from one level of care to another, she knew that families are usually in agreement and aware of the transition to long term care. This seemed uncanny. In a strange way, this was beginning to seem like the kidnapping her mother had imagined.

***

On October 10, 2017, Mara felt like she was in a one-person advocacy army, fighting with a facility and now having insurance issues. She believed that her mother could be transferred to a higher level of care if the documentation would allow for that to happen. She left a voicemail message for Iesha, the review nurse at the Alexandria rehab stating, "Hi Iesha. This is Mara, Ms. Mitchell's daughter. Can you please contact Toni at the insurance company with clinicals for acute rehab authorization and or information to get an extension at the Alexandria facility? I spoke with Toni, and she said that she would provide authorization for acute rehab if the documentation showed that my mom meets criteria. Thank you so much."

Mara tried working both angles because insurance coverage at the current rehab was about to end again based on physical and occupational therapy's documentation. Iesha returned Mara's call and said, "Hi Mara. This is Iesha. There will be a peer to peer review tomorrow. The medical director from the insurance company and the medical director from the acute rehab will discuss your mom's case and decide if she will be authorized for acute rehab."

This peer-to-peer review was because of authorization not being provided initially for the Rockville acute rehab. Should she ask the pulmonologist to speak on behalf of her mother? Based on the pulmonologist's level of participation at the care plan meeting and from his interactions with her, Mara did not believe that his input toward the peer-to-peer review would be helpful. She did not want him to ask the director of therapy for any assistance with that request.

On the following day, Mara received a call from Iesha who stated, "The acute rehab authorization was denied. The extension for your mother to remain with insurance coverage at the Alexandria facility was granted for six additional days and another peer-to-peer review would be conducted at that time."

Mara was extremely disappointed with the news about the denial of authorization to enter an acute rehabilitation facility. She was, however, grateful for the extension at the skilled nursing facility. At least her mom would have insurance coverage to continue to be there, even if it were for only six more days.

"Thanks Iesha. Fingers crossed for the next peer review to go well."

Mara wondered, is the peer-to-peer review dependent on what the Alexandria Rehab saw as financially beneficial? She could not help thinking that young people...young people in the USA, anyway, should be taught early to set aside millions for their own elderly and rehabilitation care since programs and facilities listened only to the argument of the dollar.

Chapter 40

Self-pay

Mara was very hopeful that the next peer to peer review would result in a more favorable outcome for her mother to go to the acute rehab. She tried to follow up with Iesha on the day that the authorization would expire, however, she was unable to reach her and left a voicemail message. There was no return call.

On October 18, 2017, she then followed up with Jolly, the social worker. Jolly informed her, "Authorization for your mother's continued stay here at the Alexandria rehab ended yesterday and there would be no further peer to peer review."

Mara had submitted documentation to the insurance department that conducted the reviews and included her report of the progress that her mother had made including the daily walks with her in the dining room. She realized that there could have been numerous peer-to-peer reviews, but the outcome would be the same, if the physical therapists continued to document that her mother was a long-term care candidate, despite the amount of progress that Denise had made and was continuing to make. They were the official source of information, and, in her estimation, they did not care. She knew from conversations with her mother, that her mother did not want to reside at the Alexandria facility or any nursing home. In their experience at the facility, despite whatever issues Denise was experiencing, whether it was difficulty breathing, pain or the need for assistance to the restroom, she was forced to wait for extended periods. Mara as well as Denise's other visitors, had witnessed that type of behavior numerous times. To them, it became a matter of whether to report those issues daily, as they occurred so often. What would be the incentive for Denise to continue to stay at the facility long term, when it was already unbearable for her, and she was only there for short-term rehabilitation?

The news that her mother was now considered to be a private pay patient at the facility was very disturbing. Mara felt as though the facilities did not expect or want patients to make progress. She made a number of calls as she tried to persuade someone to listen to her and to make the right decision. She called the insurance case manager Toni.

"Hi Toni. This is Mara. When you get this message can you please give me a call back regarding my mother Denise at the Alexandria rehab?" She did not get a return call.

Mara called Toni again the following day, "Hi Toni. It's Mara again. Can you please direct me to who I need to speak with regarding my mom, Denise at the Alexandria rehab? I understand that she is no longer being covered by the insurance, but I really disagree and want to appeal if I can. She has made so much progress and she really deserves a chance to reach her full potential by going to the acute rehab, especially since they have accepted her. She is walking with me, and I am trying to prevent her from becoming bedbound if she does not receive any therapy. My number is…Thanks Toni." Again, there was no return call.

Mara contacted Jolly the social worker at the rehab, "Hi Jolly, can you please tell me if there is a physiatrist who sees patients at the facility?"

Mara's hope was that there would be a physiatrist who saw patients at the facility who would conduct an independent assessment and determine that her mother was appropriate for acute rehab. That person's assessment could be submitted to the insurance for authorization to be provided. Jolly told her "No. There is no physiatrist that sees patients at the facility. If your mother needs to go out for a private appointment to be seen by one, it will need to be approved by Dr. Kulkarti."

With frustration, Mara simply replied, "Okay thanks." She wanted to have her mother transferred out of the facility but while she remained there, Mara continued to pursue therapy options. She left a voicemail message for Iesha saying, "Hi Iesha. This is Mara, Ms. Mitchell's daughter. Would you mind finding out from the insurance if they would consider covering therapy services only?"

She thought that her mother would benefit from therapy and would try to see if it would be covered, even if her boarding at the facility turned out to be private pay. She did not receive a return call from Iesha. Mara felt as though she had run out of options for requesting assistance. In this wonderful country, you had to pay for health care, and you were made to feel like a beggar if your views did not mesh with those of the official care facilities, some of which were quite uncaring. She contacted member services at the insurance company, and she was told by the representative Darian, "Your mother does not meet medical necessity to stay under skilled care at the current facility nor to be transferred elsewhere. A second level appeal could be submitted that should support why your mother needs to go to another facility." Mara was once again disappointed. She thought that it was worth a try to contact membership services. Darian's suggestion was to do the same as had been done before. The problem again would be that the therapists' documentation never changed so the response would continue to be the same, was Mara's thought.

Mara heard from Enid on her mother's job who provided her with information for a health care advocate for the employees at their workplace. Mara contacted the health care advocate, Elisa Nay, and filled her in with all that had transpired in her mother's care. Elisa was concerned. She found out more about the details and got involved with Denise's case soon after she and Mara had spoken. Mara told her mother about the health care advocate. Denise raised her eyebrows. She smiled. She closed her eyes. She opened them. She looked at her daughter. She asked, "You think she can help?" Mara said, "I hope so." She wanted to leave the facility now. She seemed particularly eager because she was no longer receiving therapy again, this time because there was no insurance coverage.

Cost of therapy

On October 19, 2017, there was a telephone call from Jolly, the social worker.

"Hi Mara. This is Jolly. I just wanted to inform you that you could inquire about the cost of therapy that you could pay privately for, here at the facility. Would you like me to get the cost from the therapy department?"

Mara was annoyed. Her response showed her annoyance. "I would not pay the therapists to pretend that they are providing therapy to my mother. The therapy department was being compensated by the insurance company and they refused to continue to work with my mom, so I do not understand their justification for providing therapy privately. What about if I got a therapist to come in to work with her?"

Jolly responded, "No. The facility does not allow other non-facility related therapists to enter the premises to provide therapy."

Mara assumed that would be the case. Still, she thought, they had a nerve!

Chapter 41

Mucus plug

On October 20th, 2017, Mara was at her mother's bedside as usual, when Denise started to have some difficulty breathing. Mara pressed the call bell and then went out to the nursing station, but no one was around. She quickly went back to her mother's room. It took approximately fifteen minutes after Mara pressed the call bell before a nursing assistant arrived—then a few more minutes later her nurse entered the room with a pulse oximetry machine. Denise's oxygen saturation was at 70%. A few nurses and a respiratory therapist arrived, and all attended to her. After several minutes, the team realized that she had a mucus plug. The inner cannula within the tracheostomy tube was clogged with mucus. Mara saw it. The respiratory therapist and the nurse looked at each other. They did not say anything. Mara seethed. They of course knew that this was negligence. They should have suctioned her earlier. Now, the therapist conducted deep suctioning. The experience was traumatic for Denise. She was sobbing after the respiratory therapist suctioned her tracheostomy. Her clothing was soaked with her blood. Shortly after Denise was cleaned by the nurses and breathing via the tracheostomy again, Mara received a call from Elisa, the healthcare advocate. She stepped out of the room while the staff dealt with her mother, and she updated Elisa on her mother's status. They both agreed that event would hopefully help with presenting a case that would allow Denise to transfer to a higher level of care, an acute rehabilitation facility. They both felt that Denise needed to be managed at a facility where the staff was prepared to respond more quickly and with expertise. Given the fact that Denise had a history of having mucus plugs since the tracheostomy was in place, Elisa and Mara discussed that staff should have been vigilant to help to prevent any more emergency situations. Denise frequently had thick mucus, Mara observed, and she realized that her mother was not always able to expectorate the mucus without intervention. As a result of Denise's thick mucus, Mara frequently requested that the nurses and respiratory therapists suction her. She explained to the nurses that she was concerned that mucus would become stagnant in her lungs, creating a reservoir for bacteria.

Mara called member services at her mother's insurance company again. The representative gave her a case number. He told her that the decision from the peer-to-peer review was upheld. He told her that the next appeal would be to the employer. Mara was starting to believe that this nightmare was never-ending.

On October 24, 2017, with her mother's permission, Mara wrote a letter that would allow Elisa Nay to speak on Denise's behalf. The letter was notarized at the facility. It read:

To Whom It May Concern:

I, Denise Mitchell of sound mind, appoint my daughter Mara Mitchell and Health Care Advocate, Elisa Nay to obtain my medical information, to discuss my medical care and to speak on my behalf for medical care issues, while I continue to receive medical care and or I am in an inpatient setting.

On this 24th day of October 2017, I hereby sign this document and declare it to be my wish.

Denise Mitchell

***

On November 1, 2017, Elisa helped Mara to collect documentation that would be needed for the next review. Mara contacted medical records at the Alexandria facility and requested documentation, as she was certain that the incident whereby her mother's oxygen saturation dropped to 70% would really help her case. She received the documentation with the respiratory therapist's notes as well as the ENT's note from the director of respiratory therapy. She read the notes from the respiratory therapist Ty and found herself creating different scenarios in her mind. She thought that Ty did not remember anything out of the ordinary on the day that her mother had a mucus plug. In Mara's mind, she considered that Ty wrote his notes hours later or he wanted to ensure that he was not blamed for the mucus plug event.

He documented that Denise had some anxiety and that her oxygen level dropped to 85%. He documented that after he spoke with Denise and she calmed down, her oxygen level returned to normal. There was no mention that he needed to deep suction her and clean her inner cannula. Mara thought, *I was there at the bedside when it occurred. The inner cannula was clogged with mucus.* But they tell lies, she thought. Does this happen in all facilities? She called the facility immediately. She brought the discrepancy to Carlton's and to Edna's attention. Carlton planned to have Ty make the correction. Ty called Mara. He told her, "I'll wait until you get here this evening so you can remind me about what happened."

Really? Mara felt as though she did not have a choice. She needed accurate notes to help build a case that her mother needed a higher level of care, such as an acute rehab. Mara arrived at her mother's room at 6pm that evening. Ty entered the room just as she walked in.

He said, "Hi. Can you come with me? I will write the note. I want to make sure that I am writing what you want me to say."

She looked at him. She did not respond. She looked at her mother. She said, "Mummy I'll be right back."

She followed Ty to the respiratory therapists' office. He sat at a computer. She stood behind him. Mara said, "I am surprised that you do not remember what happened. My mom was having some trouble breathing. I called for assistance. We waited for about fifteen minutes before anyone came. You and a few nurses eventually came. My mom's nurse checked the oxygen saturation, and it was 70%. You removed the inner cannula. It was clogged. Then you did deep suctioning. There was a lot of blood coming out of the tracheostomy. After a few minutes, her oxygen saturation went up to the nineties."

With his back to her, he said, "Okay. So, she was in respiratory distress. She desaturated to 70%. The inner cannula was cleaned. She required deep suctioning. Then her saturation increased to the nineties. Got it. I cannot change the note from that date, so I will have to say it occurred on a different day." He began to type his note. She remained standing behind. She read the note, it reflected what occurred but as he told her, he changed the date. She paused on that but was not sure how to deal with that issue. Would the different date exonerate him? Why couldn't he simply correct his note? She did not know. She was bewildered by all this double dealing. She said, "Okay thanks."

She walked out of his office. She went back to her mother's room. Mara reflected that if she were not present on the evening when her mother's oxygen saturation dropped to 70%, she would have had no argument. She would not have known. They could (and would) tell her anything. But she had been there. She thought about all the times that staff kept trying to convince Denise that she had anxiety... and medicated her for what they called "anxiety."

***

November 1, 2017: Care plan meeting

Before heading to the facility, Mara received a call from Jolly for another care plan meeting that was scheduled for that afternoon.

The dietician reported, "Your mom lost a couple more pounds. I would say that the family should continue to encourage her to eat by bringing in foods that she likes."

Dr. Kulkarti reported, "We need to figure out what the issue is in terms of your mom not tolerating being weaned from the trach."

Mara said, "Yes. Perhaps you can help us to get an appointment for her to be seen by ENT." The physician responded, "I'll see what I can do."

There were no more questions or anything else to report. Again, as she had at the end of every care plan meeting, Jolly said to Mara, "We have your mom's code status as full code. Are there any changes?"

Mara responded, "No changes. She is still full code." Jolly said, "Okay. Thank you. Have a good evening." The meeting ended.

After all the documentation was collected for her mother's case, Mara contacted the department that processed external reviews. She explained that she wanted to appeal the end of the authorization at the Alexandria facility and requested that her appeal be expedited. She really did not want her mother to continue to stay at the skilled nursing facility. The issue was that Denise had become a private pay patient and was expected to pay out of pocket. The appeals department or external review department representative told

Mara that her request would be processed in a few weeks.

A few days passed. She followed up with the external review department again. She thought, *I know they said weeks but hopefully I get a different person on the phone.* She spoke with a different representative. The representative said, "I am sorry, but your appeal will not be expedited. You will get an answer in a few weeks."

Elisa, the healthcare advocate on her mother's job, told her that after the tracheostomy was revised, she should ask the physician to send a fax requesting that the external review be expedited. Mara took her advice. In the meantime, Elisa was also contacting the external review department to assist with appealing the decision to end authorization and to request that they reconsider allowing Denise to be admitted to the acute rehab. Both Mara and Elisa made multiple attempts to try to convince anyone who would listen and was able to facilitate change. If they could, they would see that Denise had every chance to live.

As a follow-up to the ENT's initial appointment, Dr. Crompton the ENT, ordered a CT scan of Denise's neck. He phoned Mara and told her that surgery may need to be considered after the CT scan. Of course, neither Denise nor Mara wanted Denise to have surgery again. The CT scan was done. According to Dr. Crompton, there was nothing obvious above the tracheostomy tube. It could be subtle, he told her. Denise needed to be monitored closely, given her history of mucus plugs. He explained that he could not make any promises that a surgical procedure would correct the problem, but that it was worth a try.

An appointment for surgery was made for the 27th of December 2017. The Alexandria rehab made ENT referrals to Dr. Crompton's office. He was aware that Denise had become a private pay patient as Mara made sure that she mentioned to him that her mother was no longer covered by the insurance at the facility and requested some assistance in obtaining an earlier date for the procedure. She wanted to have the procedure scheduled earlier, she explained, because while her mother waited to have the procedure she was being billed for her stay at the facility.

Dr. Crompton told Mara, "I really do not have any input on the dates that are available. Talk to the scheduler to see if they can change the date." Mara responded, "Okay." She contacted the scheduler and was told December 27, 2017, was the earliest date available for her mother's procedure.

Chapter 42

Placement of the G-tube

On November 12, 2017, Mara continued to see her mother daily. Denise complained of abdominal pain and back pain. Both complaints were worrisome for Mara as she knew her mother's medical history. She spoke to her mother's nurse.

"I am really concerned about my mom continuously complaining of abdominal pain. Perhaps the gastrostomy tube is what is causing the discomfort."

Mara suspected that the tube was not in place, but her mother was eating food by mouth so at least she was not being fed via the tube. The nurse continued to listen.

Mara asked, "What about making sure the tube is in the correct place, maybe an x-ray?"

The nurse responded, "Dr. Kulkarti does not like to order x-rays."

Mara said nothing. She wondered what sense that answer made. The nurse left the room and returned shortly after. She looked at Mara. She told her that she had been advised to check for placement herself. She raised the bed to her waist level. She smiled at Denise. Denise smiled. She performed her placement check by placing a syringe at the end of the gastrostomy tube and placed a stethoscope on Denise's abdomen with the earpieces in her ear. She pushed some air through the syringe as she listened. Mara watched. She thought to herself, *well, she is using the correct technique. What could be causing the stomach pain?*

The nurse told Mara, "It is in place." She gave Denise pain medication. She pushed one of the buttons on the siderail and lowered the bed to the lowest level. She smiled at Denise. Mara said, "thank you." She looked at Mara. She smiled and said, "you're welcome." She left the room.

Mara allowed her mother to rest. They stayed in her mother's room that evening, without exercising. Denise was not feeling well and needed time to allow the medication to take effect. Mara prayed at her mother's bedside and left the facility when visiting hours ended. She sent out the usual group text messages to remind family and friends of the prayers that were needed. She believed in prayer, and she knew they did, too.

On November 13, 2017, the following morning, Mara received a phone call from her mother's nurse at the Alexandria facility. Nurse Jamila informed her, "Dr. Kulkarti told me to call to ask if you want the gastrostomy tube to be removed."

Mara was surprised. She told Jamila, "My interest is to determine the cause of the pain. I would leave the decision to remove the tube to the physician."

She did not want them to remove the tube and later learn that they had not thought that a clever idea but removed the tube at the patient's daughter's request. Later in the evening when Mara visited her mother, Jackson the assistant nurse manager and Anna, a floating nurse entered the room. Jackson spoke to Denise. She was familiar with him, but he still introduced himself and the nurse who accompanied him.

He said, "Ms. Mitchell, I am Jackson, and this is Anna. We are here to remove the gastrostomy tube from your stomach."

Denise looked up at them with raised eyebrows. He continued, "It will not be painful." She sighed. She was relieved. Her nurse had medicated her for pain at an hour and a half earlier. Jackson continued to talk to Denise as he was about to discontinue the tube, "I see you have a lot of nice greeting cards," he said. That served as a distraction, Mara realized, so that her mother would not focus on any discomfort. Good. As he removed the tube, he acknowledged, "That is why you were having pain. It was already on its way out, just resting underneath the skin in your abdomen."

Denise did not appear to have any discomfort while the tube was being pulled out. Both Denise and Mara were relieved that the tube was finally removed, especially now that they were learning that it really was the cause of the pain. So here we are again, Mara thought. What, then, was all that checking earlier to ensure that the tube was in place? Hadn't she been assured then that it was? She and her mother spent a few more minutes just enjoying each other's company. They said prayers and Mara left. She sent out updates with the usual requests for prayers.

Chapter 43

Call for help

Mara visited her mother as usual the next evening. Denise was sitting upright in the bed. She was waiting for her daughter. She knew the time that she should expect to see Mara and so did the staff. Mara walked into the room at 6pm. Denise smiled when she saw her. Mara hugged her mother. Denise told her, "I need to use the commode."

Mara pressed the call-bell. They waited for someone to respond. She asked her mother, "How was your day?"

Denise shrugged her shoulders. "Did you have a good day?" She asked Mara. Mara smiled. "It was okay" she said.

Twenty minutes went by. A nursing assistant walked into the room. He asked, "How can I help you?"

"She needs help to get to the commode." He put a pair of gloves on. He walked over to the bed. He placed his hands underneath her left arm. He said, "hold the siderail."

Denise held the rail of the bed with her right hand. "Okay stand," he said. She stood, then pivoted to the commode with his support. She sat down and smiled with relief.

"Thank you," she said. He started to walk away, then turned around.

"Call when you're finished."

He walked out of the room. Denise finished using the commode. Mara pressed the call-bell. They waited for half an hour.

"I can't sit on this any longer," Denise said to Mara, it's too uncomfortable."

Mara and Denise decided that they could manage without waiting any longer. Mara stood on her mother's left side. She placed her hand underneath her mother's left arm. Denise held on to the armrest of the commode. She lifted her buttocks off the seat of the commode. Mara helped her to stand. Denise stood upright. Her feet slid forward.

She grabbed the siderail of the bed. Mara supported her on the left side. Denise continued to slide. Mara supported her to the floor. She looked at her mother's socks.

"It is the socks. I thought you were wearing the non-skid socks. Are you okay?"

"Yes, I am okay.

Denise looked up at her daughter. Maybe somebody will come by," she said. They waited for another fifteen minutes. Bada, an older male nursing assistant, walked into the room. He did not say anything. He placed his hands underneath Denise's arms. He lifted her up. He placed her on the bed. He straightened her in the bed.

She looked up at him and said, "thank you."

"You are welcome," He responded abruptly, before leaving the room.

***

From that day on, the nurses' documentation focused on the 'fall to the floor' when Denise's daughter was helping her. Mara reflected that she had been walking daily at the facility with her mother and she had not sustained any slips or falls. She reasoned, if she had paid attention to the socks her mother was wearing, the slip to the floor could have been prevented. More than anything, though, she thought that if they had responded when her mother called, there would have been no fall. They simply did not respond when patients (or residents, as they named them) called. She felt almost helpless in this situation. *Almost,* she reminded herself. She would not let them do that to her. She was not helpless. She prayed with her mother and sent requests for prayers to friends and family.

Invoice

Later that night when Mara got home, she noticed that she had received an invoice from the facility in the mail. The bill was approximately $59,000.00 plus. Mara knew that neither she nor her mother could afford to pay that bill. A payment plan must be arranged to clear that balance. Mara sat on the couch and focused on the itemized bill. These facilities were expensive, and the insurance was no longer covering care. They did not have to be efficient to be expensive. But what had they done to accumulate this amount? As she scanned the bill, she put her right hand over her mouth. Her eyes opened wide. *Oh my God! Wait. Why is she getting a bill for the ventilator? She has been off the ventilator since September! This is November. And therapy? She has not received therapy for over a month! This bill is saying that the services were provided up to the beginning of this month,*

November? Am I missing something here? She massaged her temples. *Okay, let me go take a shower. We will deal with this tomorrow.*

***

Mara arrived at her workplace the next morning. She tried to focus on her job as the other part of her considered how to deal with the billing situation for her mother. *I need to speak with billing at the facility.* She took her cell phone out of her bag. She dialed the number for Trina, the billing specialist. Trina picked up on the second ring. She said, "This is Trina."

Mara pressed her index finger in a circular motion on her right temple. She said in a calm voice, "Hello Trina. This is Mara, Denise Mitchell's daughter." She paused.

Trina said, "Hello Mara. How can I help you?"

"I am looking at the bill that I received, and it is not accurate. My mom is not receiving therapy services. She has not been receiving those services for a while now. I also see that the ventilator is mentioned as part of respiratory services and she has been off the ventilator for almost two months."

Trina sighed audibly. Mara furrowed her eyebrows and shook her head, from one side to the other. Was she not supposed to complain if the facility was trying to make her pay for services not rendered?

Trina said, "I'll contact the respiratory, as well as the physical and occupational therapy departments to confirm that your mom is not receiving those services."

"Okay thank you. Bye." She ended the call.

A few days later, Mara received an invoice from the Alexandria Rehab via email. She sat on her couch. It read payment due, $23,000.00. She thought to herself, *so they adjusted the bill. This bill is $36,000.00 less than the first one. Ventilator? Denise had been tolerating trach collar all day until 2 am into the following day as of August 23rd, 2017 and was completely off the ventilator by September 6th, 2017. Why was the insurance also being billed for a ventilator?*

Again, that questioning person inside of Mara was busy. Is there a physician, a nurse, or person in administration at Northern Metropolitan Hospital who is interested in a safe outcome for my mother? Is there anyone at the Baltimore facility who cares or who cared? Was there anyone at the Alexandria facility interested in a safe discharge to home for my mother? Is there ever a time that the insurance representatives think about my mother as a person? Of course not, she answered herself. The medical system is about money, not about people. So, she thought, that is the system that I work in.

Worrying continuously about her mother, conscious that no facility really cared, she tried to figure out how to have her mother moved to a safer environment. Was there a safer environment in these facilities? How did one find out who was who? Personal references? Since the insurance could not be convinced that she was not safe at the Alexandria facility, Denise was now a private pay patient. Her care, Mara felt, was of even poorer quality than it had been while she had insurance coverage. She felt that she needed to identify at least one trustworthy person at the rehab who could ensure that her mother was receiving appropriate care and attention.

***

Her mother had become friends with one of the nursing assistants, Fiona. Eager to find someone who seemed trustworthy, Mara referred to Fiona as her mother's daughter at the rehab. Fiona was diligent. Even on days that she was not assigned to care for Denise, she would quickly visit to provide personal care. Both Denise and Mara appreciated her mindfulness and the time she spent with Denise overall. While the other nursing assistants and nurses were determined that Denise should use a bedpan and if not, the bedside commode, Fiona would allow Denise to use the restroom because she knew Denise wanted to have privacy when she used the bathroom, like most people would. Fiona wheeled her to the restroom with the wheelchair and assisted her to stand and then sit on the commode. This was done with the assistance of just Fiona, one person. Fiona took Denise outside of the building in front of the lobby to allow her to have fresh air. Denise was pleased. She spoke well of Fiona. One day, Fiona sent Mara a picture via text message, of her mother as they sat outside. Mara was at work. She looked at the picture. She smiled. There might not be good facilities because of the overall attitudes but there *are* good people around.

Later that evening, Mara was at her mother's bedside. She showed her the picture that she had received from Fiona. Denise frowned. She said, "I do not like it. I need a haircut. I have a lot more gray hair now. I look old! I do not even have a little lipstick." Mara looked at the picture again. She said to her mother, "Mummy, you look fine. I was so happy when I saw it. I am glad you went outside." She hugged her mother. In her mind she thought, *this picture brings so much joy to me. It's the other things I have to keep thinking about—monitoring medications that my mother is receiving, her complaints of pain, staff not suctioning her when they should, monitoring the oxygen tank when she is not in her room, therapy that I have to provide, ordering her meals, slow responses for assistance, helping my mother to the commode when I visit and billing issues.* She continued to sit at her mother's bedside. Visiting hours ended. She hugged her mother goodnight.

At work the next morning, Mara called Trina at the facility. She said, "Thanks for the adjusted bill. I would like to have a payment arrangement because I cannot afford to pay in one payment. Also, I would like to have an itemized bill." Trina responded, "I would have to get back to you on that." Mara said, "Okay thanks. Bye." They ended the call.

Chapter 44

Payment due

Despite the request for a payment plan arrangement as well as the ENT's recommendation for close monitoring, the nursing facility began to have discussions with Mara about having her mother discharged to home. Of course, Mara would have liked to have her mother home, but she was only interested in a safe discharge plan. There were too many factors to be considered. Denise would need frequent monitoring around the clock. She was unable to assist with suctioning her trach because her left hand was affected by the strokes and since care was never provided to address that hand, it would have been a challenge to manage with just the right hand. Insurance had not guaranteed that they would provide caregivers around the clock. Mara had to work, so staying home with her mother was not an option. There were too many stairs at Denise's and Mara's house that Denise would need to maneuver. She had not climbed or practiced with stairs at the rehab. The facility was not interested in whether there was a safe discharge plan or not. They wanted to be paid. They had done nothing to assist with arrangements to ensure that the insurance would have allowed Denise to continue to receive skilled care. They proceeded to make plans for training for Mara to provide care to her mother. Carlton provided tracheostomy training. The nurses monitored the administration of medications to Denise by Mara. There was no training from the therapy department. Mara had received her own training from her friends at work in the therapy department. There were so many decisions and so much to address, Mara knew that she had to sort things out. This entire business was about money, not about people. Amid all the confusion, with the realization that money was the major factor, and they did not have it, Mara tried to devise a plan. What could she do?

As usual, after her workday ended, Mara visited her mother. They spent a few minutes in her room. Mara wheeled her mother in the wheelchair out to the dining room. They ate dinner. They walked the perimeter of the dining room. Mara could see that her mother had made significant improvement. If only the insurance company would send a representative to conduct their own assessment, she thought. They would see that she had improved enough to be given a chance for acute rehabilitation. Just one more facility, she thought, one that could take her—and hopefully an acute rehabilitation facility, and then she could be home.

After they walked, they went back to Denise's room. They looked at homes for sale on-line. They saw quite a few houses that piqued their interest. While there, at her mother's bedside, Mara emailed a few of the agents for more information.

Denise was now just awaiting the laryn-goscopy and bronchoscopy in the operating room. It was to determine if there was a blockage in her air-way. The Fairfax Hospital scheduled the procedure on December 27th, 2017. Mara was worried. She reflected; this is November. My mother is now pri-vate pay. While at work, she called Carlton, the di-rector of respiratory services at the rehab. She asked that he and Dr. Kulkarti, assist in obtaining an ear-lier appointment for her mother's procedure.

Carlton called Mara later in the day. He told her that he had not been successful in getting an earlier appointment. Her mother's friend Ali provided Mara with the contact information of an

ENT, Dr. Terry, who would be able to assist. Mara contacted Dr. Terry. He was very empathetic. He had not practiced at the Fairfax Hospital where the procedure was scheduled to take place, in quite some time but had connections who may be able to assist and get the procedure scheduled earlier. He provided Mara with the contact information of one of his colleagues, Dr. Shah. Mara spoke with Dr. Shah who was willing to investigate the case. He said he would get back to Mara about his decision. It was all a waiting game at that point. The next correspondence that Mara received from the nursing facility was another copy of the bill for the almost $24,000.00. Mara had requested a payment arrangement but had not heard anything about it. They were demanding payment.

***

Mara was at her desk at work. She received a phone call from Jolly, the social worker at the facility. Jolly said, "You would have to list your mom's house for sale. She has a bill here at the facility and that needs to be paid. It may not even get sold but we must see that it is listed."

Mara listened. She thought to herself, *why is she telling me this?* Furious, she responded, "I am not putting my mother's house for sale. That is the same house that she is looking forward to returning to. It would break her heart. Plus, I do not have the authority to sell her house."

She could hear her own voice getting louder. She got up from her desk and walked briskly down the hallway. Mara held the phone to her ear. Silence. Neither of them said anything. Mara got to the double doors and walked out of the nursing unit so she could have privacy for the call. Jolly was still on the line.

"Okay, Mara" she said. "I will let you think about it. Bye."

Mara stared out the window of the waiting area on the unit.

"Okay, bye," she said. Mara put the phone in the pocket of her lab coat. What should she do? She closed her eyes.

Chapter 45

Respiratory distress

On November 20, 2017, Mara was at her hospital in Germantown, walking out of a patient's room. Her cell phone rang in her pocket. She quickly looked at it. It was someone from the Alexandria facility. She answered, "Hello." She walked toward the exit on the unit.

A soft voice, "Hello. Is this Mara?"

Mara took a deep breath. She said, "yes, this is Mara." The person on the other end cleared her throat. She said, "this is Beatrice, one of the nurses at the Alexandria Rehab. Your mom had syncope and she vomited four times today. We transferred her to the Alexandria hospital."

Mara sat down on one of the chairs in the waiting area. She leaned forward. Both of her elbows were resting on her knees. The phone was in her left hand.

"What was she doing?" She asked. "Was someone helping her to the commode, and she felt dizzy or fainted?"

"No. She was sitting in her bed. She just started to vomit."

"I wonder what made her vomit. Did she eat something different?"

"No. I don't think so."

"Okay. Thanks for letting me know Beatrice."

Mara put her cell phone in her pocket. She said to herself, *I wonder what caused her to get sick. The nurse does not seem to have much information.* Should she try to leave work to see her mother? She would have to talk to her manager. She took the phone out of her pocket. She looked at the time. It was four thirty in the afternoon, half hour before her workday ended. *Oh, well there is no point in trying to leave early.* She stood. She took a deep breath. She started to walk back to the nursing station. *What else do I have to do before I get out of here? Ughh. I have some more charting to do.* She began to walk fast. She sat at her desk. She began to type. Several minutes passed. She looked at the time on her computer. It was 5pm. She shut her computer down and picked up her bag. Her mother was on her mind. *I hope she is okay*, she thought to herself. She began to walk quickly toward the exit. The elevator door was already open. She stepped in and pressed the button for the first floor. She hurried out of the elevator on the first floor and walked briskly to the parking lot. Mara sat in her car. She took a deep breath. She sat back with her head against the headrest for a couple of minutes. She turned on the ignition. She drove out of the parking lot and headed toward the highway. The traffic was heavy on 270S but was moving steadily. She turned up the volume to listen to the soca cd that was already in the player. After about a forty-five-minute drive, Mara turned onto the hospital parking lot in Alexandria Virginia.

She walked to the emergency room entrance. There was a security officer sitting at the desk. He was African American, in his mid-twenties. He smiled. She signed the clipboard at his desk. He handed her a visitor's badge. He told her, "It's the first room on your right." She walked toward the direction that he told her. She saw her mother through the glass doors.

Denise was lying on a stretcher. Her head was elevated at about a forty-five-degree angle. Her eyes were closed. Mara sat quietly on the chair next to the stretcher. A physician walked in shortly after she arrived. He was Caucasian, about 5ft 11in tall. He was in his mid-fifties. He kept both his hands inside the pockets of his lab coat. He walked closer to Mara.

He smiled, "Are you, her daughter?" Mara looked up at him. "Yes, I am Mara" she said. He took a deep breath. He looked over at Denise with a concerned expression. Her eyes were still closed.

"I'm Dr. Johnson," he said to Mara. "Your mom had a mucus plug at the nursing home. We did some suctioning and had to give her more support with the ventilator. Right now, she is on full vent support. The machine is doing the work of breathing for her. We will keep an eye on her. Once there is a bed upstairs, she will be transferred up there."

Mara looked over at her mother. She looked back at the physician, "okay, thank you" she said. He walked out of the room.

She continued to sit next to her mother. She thought about what the physician had just told her. She reflected, *She had a mucus plug? Why is this happening? She has a smaller tracheostomy now. The nurses and respiratory therapists at the rehab know this. They need to suction her frequently. She has a tough time getting rid of the mucus by herself because the trach size is so small. I have seen her struggle with it. Staff have been in the room when it happens. If they would suction her at the rehab as they should, she would not need to be hospitalized for this. It is as though they allow the mucus to become stagnant, while exposing her to become sick. I wonder if the staff at the rehab cannot identify when there is a mucus plug.* And the worrying thought, *they just do not care. They know that she will get clogged up and become ill, but they cannot be bothered.*

Dr. Johnson and a caucasian man in his thirties walked into the room. The young man said, "hi" as he walked behind Mara. She glanced up at him and read the title on his shirt, 'respiratory therapist.' She said, "hi." She moved her chair away from the stretcher.

The physician spoke to Denise, "Ms. Mitchell, we'll try to change your breathing tube here."

Denise's eyes remained closed. Dr. Johnson and the therapist attempted to change the type of tracheostomy. They struggled. Denise opened her eyes. There was blood on her neck. She closed her right fist. She hit the stretcher with her right hand. Dr. Johnson said, "okay we'll stop." He turned to Mara.

"The ostomy in her neck, is already closing," he said. "Its size has decreased and the trach we were trying to put in is too large for the space."

Mara nodded. She looked at her mother laying on the stretcher. She was saddened to see her mother having so much discomfort. She began to think, *oh, so if this trach stays in place, mummy could have the same problem again at the rehab. She cannot be on the vent forever. She will not!* Her anxiety level started to increase. She thought about the nurses and therapists at the rehab. *I do not know if they will change how they provide care to her.* The therapist wiped the blood from Denise's neck with gauze. The physician held Denise's hand, "hang in there" he said.

He walked out of the room. The therapist walked over to the trash can. He dumped the gauze in it. He turned. He looked at Mara. He said, "take care" and walked out.

So, what now? What did one do? Just nothing?

A few minutes later, the nurse walked in. She wore her hair in a ponytail. She was blonde, in her early twenties. She wore dark blue scrubs. She had a bright smile. She said, "we got a bed upstairs." The therapist walked back in. He placed a small monitor on the bed. He disconnected the overhead monitor and attached everything to the monitor that he had placed on the bed. The nurse told Mara, "You can come with us." They wheeled Denise out of the room and headed to the elevator. Denise was transferred to the step-down unit on the second floor of the hospital. Mara recognized some of the staff from her mother's previous admission. She waited outside of the room while they settled her mother in the room.

After several minutes, one of the nurses came to door, "you can come in" she said to Mara. Her mother's nurse said, "My name is Ana. This is the call bell. If she needs anything while you are here, press the red button."

She pointed to the white board on the wall in the front of the room. She said, "this is my number. Visiting hours are from 9am to 9pm."

Mara said, "thank you Ana." The nurses and therapist left the room. She sat on the chair next to her mother's bed. She did not say anything. She held her mother's left hand. Denise's eyes remained closed. It was now 9pm. Mara said a silent prayer. She kissed her mother on the forehead. She left the room. She walked down the hallway to the elevator. The door was open. She took it down to the first floor. It was dark outside. She hurried to her car in the parking lot. She quickly got in her car and drove off. As she drove out of the Alexandria Hospital parking lot, she could not help thinking about her mother. *Poor mummy is going through so much. Lord will you please help?* Traffic on 395 was moving quickly. She accelerated, putting her foot lower on the gas. She kept looking in the rearview mirror. It was a long day, and she was ready to get home. About thirty minutes later she was in her driveway in Germantown, Maryland.

At her desk at work the next morning, Mara called to speak with her mother's nurse. A very friendly voice answered the phone, "Good morning! Two west. How can I help you?"

The female voice on the other end sounded very cheerful. So unusual! Mara smiled. She said, "Can I speak with the nurse for Ms. Mitchell in 2523A. This is her daughter, Mara."

The woman responded, "Sure. Hold for Sue. Have a lovely day." The call was transferred, and Sue picked up, "This is Sue." Mara answered, "Hi Sue. This is Mara, Denise Mitchell's daughter."

"Oh hi! How are you?"

"I am well thanks. Just wondering how my mom is doing."

"She is doing okay. Her vitals are stable. Her blood pressure was a bit high earlier, but she got something for it and seems to be doing okay. The respiratory therapist was in to see her, and they have already started to wean her from the vent."

"Oh, that's great." She thought to herself, *this seems like deja vu.* She said, "Please tell her that I called, and I'll see her later on today after work."

"Sure. I'll tell her. See you later."

It was a busy day at work for Mara. To her, the time went by quickly. At five in the afternoon, she shut down her computer. She picked up her bag and walked down the long hallway. There was no one in the hallway. She took the elevator to the first floor. She waved good evening to Leanne at the front desk. She sat in her car and rubbed her forehead. After a few minutes, she started her drive to Alexandria Hospital. Traffic was moving smoothly on 270 south. The other side, 270 north, was slow. She thought to herself, *I hope it will not be like that when I am coming back.* After about a thirty-five-minute drive, she drove into the hospital parking lot in Alexandria. She took the first vacant space near the entrance. She walked to the front desk. She presented her identification card to the security at the desk. He handed her a visitor's badge. She walked up the escalator toward her mother's unit. As she entered the room, she saw her mother sitting upright in the bed. Denise smiled. Mara walked closer to the bed and gave her mother a hug.

Before they had a chance to talk, the physician walked in. Judging from his features, making the quick assessment that she had become used to doing, she described him to herself as Ethiopian, about 5ft 8in with a protruding abdomen. He had a bright smile on his face. He looked at Mara, then at Denise. He said, "Is this your daughter?"

Denise smiled and nodded. He turned to Mara, "I am Dr. Gebrin. She's doing very well. I expect she will be discharged by Friday of this week. We are just monitoring the labs and making sure that everything is okay before we transfer her back to the nursing home. In the meantime, the therapists are weaning her from the vent. Do you have any questions?"

Mara was pleased to hear that her mother was doing well. She said, "I'd like her to be seen by an Ear Nose and Throat (ENT) physician while she's here." Dr. Gebrin's expression changed to one that Mara thought was concern.

He said, "ENT only comes in to see patients for emergencies. She will have to follow up as an outpatient."

Mara sighed. Dr. Gebrin walked toward the door, "Okay take care."

The day suggested for discharge was on Friday, November 24, 2017. That would be the day after Thanksgiving. There is a pattern here, Mara could not help thinking. Her mother had been admitted at the Northern Metropolitan Hospital on the day after Thanksgiving the previous year. Lord, she prayed, give us something to be especially thankful for.

In the days that followed, Mara went back and forth between her job at the hospital in Germantown, Maryland her home in Germantown, Maryland and the hospital in Alexandria, Virginia. Her mother continued to improve. It was now three days since she had been admitted. She was eating by mouth with no apparent issues. As Thanksgiving approached, Mara knew that she would spend the evening with her mother. Mara was scheduled to work and had planned on being with Denise after work. A few of her mother's friends had invited her to dinner but she did not feel comfortable celebrating the holiday without her mother. This was a time she usually spent with Denise, and it simply would not feel right.

Her mother's friend, Mena, invited Mara to come to her house after work to pick up food for herself and for her mother. Mara drove to Burtonsville, Maryland and picked up two bags from Aunt Mena. She was incredibly grateful. She knew that her mother would be pleased as well. She then drove to the hospital in Alexandria, Virginia to have Thanksgiving dinner with Denise. Aunt Mena, thought Mara, was highly organized. The bags contained everything—utensils, napkins, glasses, and a bottle of sparkling cider. Denise opened her eyes in amazement. She smiled. As Mara removed the contents of the bag, Denise opened her mouth and eyes wider. She kept smiling. In addition to Mena's food, Denise had also received food from Cathy. It had been a year since she was away from home and had not had a home-cooked meal such as that one. There was turkey, stuffing, mashed potato, green beans, macaroni and cheese, candied yams, ham, cornbread, cranberry sauce, pumpkin pie, and West Indian black cake. Denise said, "Mara, this is very good. Make sure you tell both, thanks for me. I am tired of eating that food at the rehab."

Mara had asked the hospital if their ENT specialist could examine her mother while she was there. It could not happen, she was told. The covering physician said an ENT specialist would only be called in for emergencies. Mara reminded herself that her mother was now a private paying patient. Was this about money again? People without vast resources were not easily recognized as emergencies. Nothing made sense... or it all did if you recognized that those who had and those who did not have meant different things when they talked about health care. She wondered how to make it clear that this was an emergency.

On the day after Thanksgiving, Denise was transferred back to the Alexandria rehab. While Mara was at her mother's side at the rehab, Dr. Kulkarti visited the room.

He said to Denise, "How are you feeling?" She responded, "I feel okay." He then turned to Mara and asked, "Was she seen by ENT at the hospital?" Mara responded, "No. I was told that they only come in for emergencies."

Dr. Kulkarti continued, "Did you ask for her to be seen by ENT?" Mara replied, "Yes, I did and that was the response that I got." Dr. Kulkarti said, "If I had known that you wanted her to be seen by ENT at the hospital, I would have contacted them."

Mara was surprised and annoyed by his comments. He was the pulmonologist and attending physician. Yet he had not checked but had left it up to her to figure out the type of care and consultants that her mother needed. Was this again that system that focused so much on money? Would those who had automatic unconditional health care built into their existence somehow have the treatment she was now struggling to ensure for her mother? What was even more puzzling to her was the fact that Dr. Kulkarti was now initiating this conversation. Had he heard something? Was he just looking for something to say? Mara recalled that prior to that last hospital's admission, at the care plan meeting on November 1st, 2017, she had asked him directly and she had also asked the director of respiratory therapy for assistance with the ENT appointment. As a follow-up, her mother's friend Cathy had also made attempts to contact Dr. Kulkarti so that he could speak with Mara. He had not responded. So, what was this about now? Was he trying to ensure that he could be said to have asked? Perhaps not, but her experience with the facility made her suspicious.

The days went by. Denise continued at the facility as a private care patient. Mara scrutinized each bill and tried to figure out what might be done if this continued. Denise's friends brought meals for her and that gave her some comfort. Sometimes, the friends called in advance and asked Mara what her mother would want to eat. Mara would then ask her mother. Denise had some sense of comfort as she placed her orders. She was excited to eat some of the foods that she had not eaten in what seemed like ages.

In circumstances that were far from routine, they tried to develop routine. Denise's friend Fannie and her daughter Sharon visited her at the rehab and gave her a much-needed haircut. Denise was pleased. She obviously enjoyed the compliments on her new hairstyle. Prior to being hospitalized, she had maintained a low haircut. While at the facility, her hair had grown a little more than she would normally allow it to, so the visit from her hairstylist friends was timely and appreciated. When they left that Saturday, leaving mother and daughter alone together, Denise said, "Mara, I want to go home. Let me go home for the weekend. I am so tired of feeling confined in this place. I need a change. I miss my house."

Denise became very tearful. She had a frown on her face. She was sitting upright in the bed. She leaned forward. She gazed down at the bed. Her right hand supported her forehead. Mara could understand that it must be difficult for her mother.

Mara explained, "Mummy I would love to take you home, but I cannot because you still have the trach. For you to be at home, more preparations need to be made including having sufficient supplies at home as well as continuous monitoring."

Denise was still unable to use her left hand as it was not addressed at the facilities and the fingers had become contracted. As a result, she was not able to assist in her own care with the trach. That meant that Mara would need to be on alert the entire time in the event her mother needed to be suctioned or to have the inner cannula cleaned. She knew that if she allowed her mother to go home with her, she would not be able to convince her that she had to return to the facility. Denise became very emotional. She wanted to go home. She began to sob. Mara embraced her mother. She said, "Come. Let us look at Trevor Noah."

She picked up her iPad and searched for Trevor Noah on YouTube. They watched a performance by the comedian on her iPad. Denise laughed. They ended their evening with prayers. Mara said, "Let's say the Lord's prayer."

They both said, "Our Father, who art in heaven, hallowed be thy name. Thy kingdom come. Thy will be done. On earth as it is in heaven. Give us this day our daily bread and forgive us our trespasses. As we forgive those who trespass against us. And lead us not into temptation but deliver us from evil. Amen." Mara embraced her mother. She kissed her on the cheek.

She said, "Sleep well." Denise smiled. She said, "Get home safe."

Chapter 46

ENT

On November 28, 2017, at four fifty-five in the afternoon, Mara was at her desk at work. She was preparing to shut down her computer. Her cell phone rang in her pocket. She immediately answered, "hello."

The male voice on the other end said, "Hi. This is Dr. Shah. You called my office a few days ago."

Mara recognized the name. He was an ear, nose, and throat specialist. She had been referred to him by Dr. Terry. He told her, "I would like to see your mother in my office tomorrow. I can see her at the Lake Ridge, Virginia location. You will need to call the office to schedule an appointment. Okay. Take care. See you tomorrow." He hung up. Mara smiled. Are prayers being answered? He said Lake Ridge. That is far. That is okay, she thought. She wanted her mother to be seen sooner than the late

December date that she was given for a procedure. It was already late in the evening. Would she be able to reach anyone at the doctor's office? She picked up her lunch bag and handbag. She walked down the hallway to the exit. She dialed the number to Dr. Shah's office. The phone rang several times. There was no answer. *I'll call first thing in the morning.*

November 29, 2017, at eight thirty the next morning, Mara contacted Dr. Shah's office and was able to get an appointment for her mother to be seen by the ENT at five o'clock that evening. She immediately contacted the Alexandria rehab to inform her mother's nurse about the appointment. Mara was told that the manager would have to call her back because she was at a meeting. As the time was passing, Mara kept looking at the clock as she had not received a phone call from the manager. She called the facility again and was placed on hold for several minutes. Finally, Edna, the unit manager came on the line.

She said, "This is Edna! How can I help you?" Her voice was very loud. Mara moved the phone away from her ear.

"Hi Edna. This is Mara, Denise Mitchell's daughter. I know this is late notice, but my mom got an appointment to see an ENT this afternoon…"

Edna immediately responded, "Yes, it is! She cannot go!"

Is that how families are generally treated? Mara thought to herself, *she is clearly angry. Why? I do not understand the attitude.* The alternative would be to have her mother wait for another month while being charged by the facility, just waiting for an ENT procedure. She had conversations about having her mother seen by an ENT quite a few times. She requested assistance from Dr. Kulkarti, the director of respiratory therapy, Carlton, and Dr. Gebrin at the Alexandria Hospital to have an earlier ENT appointment. Now, she had been able to obtain one herself. Edna told her, "Your mother would not be able to go to that appointment because I do not have a nurse to accompany her! There is a lot involved here! Transportation would have to be arranged. Who is going to arrange transportation?"

That did not sound impossible to Mara. She told Edna, "Can you please do what you can to assist? My mother is private pay and must wait until the end of December if she misses this appointment."

Edna responded, "I hear what you are saying but I am sorry, I cannot help you! A nurse will have to go with her. Where am I to get the nurse who must go with your mother? Plus, there is the issue of transportation! You will have to talk to the Director of Nursing!"

Mara responded, "Okay. What is her number?" Edna provided the number to the Director of Nursing.

Edna probably did not expect that Mara would agree to contact the director of nursing. Perhaps, in Edna's mind, the director of nursing was one to be feared by all. Well, Mara thought, I do not have the same relationship that Edna has with the director of nursing, who must be her supervisor. Mara understood that it was last minute notice to the facility, but she also sensed the lack of compassion from the nurse manager on the unit as well as from other personnel at the facility.

Mara placed a call to the director of nursing. There was no response. She left a voicemail message, "Good morning, Theresa. My name is Mara. My mother is Denise in room 101B at the facility. I need some assistance please. She has an appointment this afternoon with an ENT that was difficult to obtain, and I was told by the manager on the unit that my mother would not be able to go to the appointment because of staffing and transportation. I realize that it is last minute, but I just got the appointment today. Can you please assist? My number is…. Thank you."

She put the phone down. She looked at the time on the computer. It was twelve thirty in the afternoon. Her mother's appointment is at five. She began to tap her desk with her fingers. She checked the ringer on her phone. It was on. What should she do? She was at work. She did not want to lose track of the time and forget to follow-up. She phoned her mother's friend Breana. She needed to get support and reassurance that she was doing what was right. Her aunt Breana advised her to wait and if there was no response, then she may have to reschedule her mother's appointment. Breana tried to understand the facility's dilemma as they would find it difficult to plan with such short notice. Mara listened to her aunt's advice but also decided to send an email to the director. She would check her email faster than she would check her voicemail. She copied the facility's administrator on the email, hoping that someone would respond.

Good morning, Theresa,

I just left you a voicemail message. My mother was just scheduled for an ENT appointment at 5pm today in Lake Ridge, VA; however, I was told by the manager on the unit that she is unable to assist me.

I transfer patients to Alexandria rehab and I am realizing first-hand what my patients may be experiencing.

My mom has a follow up appointment on 12/27 for an ENT visit. She has been sitting waiting for this appointment and in the meantime continues to be private pay. I was lucky to get today's appointment. I am requesting that you please assist in allowing her to have this appointment today rather than encourage private pay cost to accumulate waiting for a later appointment.

Thank you for your time.

Mara

Shortly after this, Mara received a call from the director. The director said, "I am sorry I missed your call. I just saw your email. You would be hearing from the unit manager shortly."

Within minutes, Mara received a call from Edna. She told Mara, "Annie has graciously volunteered to go to the appointment with your mother. So go ahead and make the transportation arrangement and call us back."

Mara worked in Maryland and was not familiar with transportation companies in Virginia. For the one company that she was familiar with in Maryland, she knew they were allowed to drop off patients in Virginia; however, they did not pick up patients in Virginia. Mara called another transportation company in Maryland that provided her with a list of companies in Virginia. After making a few calls to locate a transportation company in Virginia, Mara arranged her mother's transportation for the appointment. She called the facility and provided them with the information. Mara met her mother and Annie at the rehab to accompany them to the appointment. She was disappointed as it was supposed to be a wheelchair van; however, the transport company had sent a large SUV. It was too late to make any changes. They managed to assist Denise into the truck and proceeded to the ENT's office. On the way to the appointment, Mara found herself in an odd conversation with the nurse who, to her, clearly had no facts but attempted to provide advice. Annie initiated the conversation.

She told Mara, "You should let the facility know what you need them to do in terms of scheduling appointments and they would take care of appointments for your mother."

Mara listened but did not respond. She felt as though there was so much more than simply the scheduling of appointments, that she needed the facility to take responsibility for but continuously expressing her mother's needs and expectations seemed pointless to her, especially in a conversation with someone who had no information about the circumstances. Tired, frustrated, anxious about her mother and the lack of support from the facility, Mara decided not to waste time having a conversation with Annie. It would not help. Annie did not know details.

They arrived at the doctor's office and soon after arriving Denise was seen by the male office nurse who did the intake process to collect information. The young man was very polite.

He asked the usual questions, "What is your name? Date of birth? Reason for this visit?" Denise's voice was not audible as she was not on the vent and did not use the passy-muir speaking valve. Denise mouthed her name to him while she showed him her identification band and both Mara and Annie responded to the other questions. He then asked, "Any allergies?"

Annie promptly responded, "no known allergies." Mara responded, "my mother is allergic to heparin, ARBs, ace inhibitors, Percocet, fentanyl, iodine and sulfur."

She did not bother to look at what she thought would be a ridiculous expression on Annie's face, as there had to be one. Mara was relieved that she was present for the appointment because that nurse was clueless. Mara could not imagine what type of insane joke the Alexandria rehab was making but she saw nothing funny about gambling with her mother's life.

Denise, Mara, and the rehab's nurse, all went into the examination room where the ENT saw Denise. Dr. Shah, a Middle Eastern man in his late forties, about 5ft 9in, average build, a full beard and a broad smile entered the room. The scribe, a young Caucasian man in his twenties with a low haircut, slim build, about 5ft 7in, also with a smile on his face, followed the doctor into the room. Dr. Shah, with a calm voice, introduced himself and the scribe. He proceeded to examine Denise. She was clearly afraid as she was not sure what to expect. She looked at him, then she looked at Mara. She looked at him again. At the end of the examination, he suggested that Denise should be closely monitored and would benefit from a laryngoscopy. The visit summary was provided to Mara. It read:

Unspecified tracheostomy complication

Notes: Patient with tracheotomy required following prolonged intubated following aortic surgery. On scoping she has subglottic stenosis that is partially soft. There is an airway with a 4mm tube in place. There is some component of laryngomalacia as well. She will require laryngoscopy with removal of subglottic soft stenosis with decannulation. She should be ok, but I am concerned the ostomy tube is too small and there is a risk of mucus plugging and she must stay in a setting where she can be monitored while she has it. Will discuss with current ENT, Dr. Crompton, and plan to see if earlier procedure time would be possible.

After the examination, Denise was assisted back to the truck, and they headed back to the Alexandria rehab.

Dr. Shah's office contacted the original ENT. The two physicians decided that the first ENT, Dr. Crompton, would perform the procedure two weeks earlier than the original date that had been provided to Mara. The new date for the procedure was December 12, 2017. Both Denise and Mara were nervous about the procedure but knew that it was worth a try. Neither of them wanted Denise to remain with the tracheostomy permanently and were determined to get answers so that she could move forward.

***

On December 8, 2017, as the date of the procedure approached, Mara realized that she was excited as well as nervous for her mother. She was on her way to visit her mother—earlier in the day than usual. It was her day off from work. She was driving south on 270. Her phone rang. She used Bluetooth. She answered. It was the pre-surgical nurse Bonnie, at the Fairfax hospital. Bonnie had some questions to ask Mara. She was completing a questionnaire regarding Denise. The questionnaire consisted of routine questions such as identifying information for Denise, allergies, past and present medical history, and any other pertinent information.

"So, I understand your mother has a feeding tube," Bonnie said.

"No, she had a feeding tube, but it was discontinued."

"No. The nurse at the Alexandria rehab Annie, specifically said that your mother has a feeding tube and that they're flushing it every shift."
Mara took a breath. She said, "Ms. Bonnie. My mother had a feeding tube but no longer has one. I was with her until 9 o'clock last night and she did not have a feeding tube. Unless they inserted one after I left, which I highly doubt, she does not have one. They would have had to get consent and they do not insert feeding tubes at the rehab, which means that they would have had to transfer her to the hospital to have a feeding tube placed. My mother does not have a feeding tube."
Mara realized that her response was so verbose that Bonnie could have said, 'okay, I got it,' however, Bonnie simply responded, "Okay thank you."

Mara had been present on November 13, 2017 when the feeding tube was discontinued. This was almost a month later. Mara thought, *if I needed more evidence, I have it. I am on my own. The facility is not interested. In fact, they could be dangerous. I do not know how I am going to do it in such an unsupportive system, but I need to have my mother transferred to another skilled nursing facility, even if it is without insurance coverage.*

Mara figured perhaps she could make payments to the Alexandria facility and, in the meantime, get her mother to a place where her needs would be met. She asked Jolly to send her mother's clinical documentation to Lory Alden. They had previously accepted her mother and Mara hoped that they would have availability for her this time. Jolly agreed to send the information. Mara contacted the admissions director at Lory Alden, Sara, to express interest in having her mother transferred to that facility. Sara indicated that she would consider accepting Denise and advised Mara to have the Alexandria facility send the clinical documentation to her. Mara had already done so. She followed up with Jolly.

"Hi Jolly, it is Mara. I'm just following up on the status of the clinicals being sent to Lory Alden."

"I have not had a chance to send the clinicals," Jolly replied.

"Do you think you will be able to send it this afternoon? They are expecting it."

"I'll try." Mara realized that she would have to continuously remind Jolly that she needed the information to be sent. She considered requesting her mother's information from medical records and sending them to Lory Alden herself but that was not protocol. The facility would not accept the information from her. Still, she did not know this to be a fact. Perhaps she could try? There was a lot happening, a lot for her to process. How could she get information and make decisions about so many different things? She would have to try.

Chapter 47

Bullying

On December 11, 2017, the day prior to Denise's procedure, Mara walked into her mother's room at the Alexandria rehab. Denise was awake and smiled when she saw Mara. The ambu bag, the device used to deliver oxygen when a patient was not breathing or not breathing adequately, was on Denise's bed next to her. She was wearing her eyeglasses which she wore mostly to read. Mara glanced around the room and noticed that there was a letter on her mother's bedside table. The window blind was down, and the overhead light was on.

Mara asked her mother, "Did they use that on you today?" She was referring to the ambu bag. Denise responded, "Yes. Last night." Mara realized that that did not make sense because if it had been used the previous night, it probably would not have still been on the bed. She knew that her mother had difficulty determining if it was day or night when the blind in the window was down. Curiously, perhaps, she could be quite capable of hiding from Mara details that could upset her. Even though Mara had asked the nurses to keep the blind up during the daytime, unless they were providing personal care, so that her mother could be oriented with time, her request had been completely ignored. Mara picked up the letter on the bedside table. It read:

Dear Mara Mitchell and Denise Mitchell

On November 27, 2017, our finance office sent you a letter requesting payment made on the Account#22222 for Denise Mitchell. In addition, our finance department has had several conversations with you concerning acceptable payment being made on this account. To date, you have failed to make full payment of the past due balance on this account. Your failure to pay this amount owed as required and agreed has forced us to initiate discharge proceedings.

This letter is provided to you to serve as your 30-day Official Notice of Discharge. On January 11, 2018, you will be discharged from Alexandria rehab to your care for "Breach of Contract" due to non-payment. You will be discharged to Germantown address with home health services or to a nursing facility of your choice of which we will assist you in transferring.

Prior to sending this letter of discharge to you, a discussion took place with Dr. Kulkarti (the attending physician) and in conjunction with the Assistant Administrator of Nursing and resident's social worker to minimize the effects of the discharge and to determine the care and kind of services that you shall require upon the transfer. I suggest that you aid in this process.

Alexandria rehab stands ready to provide preparation and orientation to you to insure a safe and orderly transfer from the facility. You may contact me or your Social Worker at Alexandria rehab to locate and coordinate services needed for a smooth transition. It is understood that you have the right to choose your own service providers.

Mara was furious. How could they do this? Hadn't she only recently talked to them about a transfer? Was this what health care was like in this wonderful place? Was there no interest in the individual? She had even asked Trina from the finance department about a payment plan for the bill of $23,000.00, and there had been no response. Were all facilities like this? They wanted the entire amount in one payment. As she looked at the letter, the director of respiratory therapy entered the room.

Mara said to him, "Can you tell me why this is sitting here?" She was referring to the ambu bag. He responded, "Your mom had some anxiety."

Mara then stated, "I would hate to find out that..." Carlton continued, "I am telling you. It was anxiety." Of course, Mara thought! Her mother must have read the letter. If so, it would have been very scary and upsetting for her.

Mara tried her best not to show any other emotion than she already had when she spoke with Carlton. She did not want to upset her mother any further. Her role was to provide as much support as she could for her mother, especially with the up-coming procedure that Denise was nervous about. Before she left, they watched Trevor Noah again until Denise got tired.

Mara prayed, "Lord, we thank you for all that you've done for us. We come to you again to ask for your mercy as mummy gets ready for a procedure tomorrow. We ask that you keep her safe in the hands of her caregivers. Give her faith. Bless all those who care for her. Give them all that they need. We know that nothing is impossible for you. We thank you for hearing our prayers. This we ask in Jesus' name. Amen."

She sent out an update via text message:

Hello everyone, mummy is scheduled to have a procedure to-morrow to help with the weaning from the trach. Continued prayers are very much appreciated.

She hugged her mother. She stood. She said, "Think pleasant thoughts mummy. Sleep well.

I will see you tomorrow." Denise attempted to smile. She said, "get home safe."

Laryngoscopy and bronchoscopy

December 12, 2017, the next day, Mara met her mother along with one of the nurses from the Alexandria facility at the Fairfax hospital. Denise and the rehab's nurse were already in the pre-operative area. Mara was invited to go in to wait with them until it was time for surgery. She got to the pre-operative area and her mother was sitting on a stretcher in one of the rooms. As usual, she smiled when she saw her daughter, but she was obviously nervous and cold. The hospital's nurse was very pleasant but did not say much. The rehab's nurse was also pleasant. She left and returned shortly after with a warm blanket for Denise. The procedure was to determine if and where there was a blockage in Denise's airway and to remove excess tissue. Dr. Crompton met them in the pre-operative area and spoke with them briefly. Shortly after meeting the physician, preparations were made to take Denise into the operating room. Mara said a quick prayer.

"Thank you, Lord, for mummy. Please let everything go well for her. Keep her safe."

"I'll be in the waiting area, waiting for you," Mara told her mother. She kissed her on the cheek. Denise was wheeled away in the direction of the operating room.

Mara and the nurse from the Alexandria rehab went out into the waiting area. They sat separately, allowing each other privacy. Mara had not eaten before she got there, so she ate her sandwich and fruits and waited patiently. She prayed silently, asking for a good outcome with her mother's procedure. After a few hours, Dr. Crompton appeared. He updated Mara.

He told her, "Well, everything went well. Your mom would have some pain, but it should not be a significant amount of pain. Her throat would be sore, and she would have some bleeding from the tracheostomy. The rehab would be able to start plugging the tracheostomy or at least attempt to wean her from it in a couple of days. She is in the recovery room. The nurses would allow you both to go back to see her when she is settled, and they are ready."

Mara did not realize how scared she had been until after she had seen her mother's surgeon. She knew that her mother was having the procedure under anesthesia and just that fact was a bit worrisome. After the conversation with the doctor, Mara decided to focus on her next task. She sent out a text message:

Hello everyone, surgery went well. My mom will soon be on her way back to Alexandria Rehab.

     She sat there in the waiting area and drafted a letter to the administration at the Alexandria facility. Prior to her mother's procedure, she knew that she could not focus on a response but now that was behind her, she needed to address some issues with the facility. The letter was addressed to the administrator, the director of nursing, the social worker, and the billing specialist. The letter read:

Good afternoon,

I received the discharge notice that was left in my mother's room. Alexandria rehab has my address as I see it listed in the letter; however, it was decided to hand-deliver to my mother's bedside on the day prior to her having surgery; very insensitive and a form of bullying. The ambu bag was on my mother's bed when I arrived yesterday. She has anxiety and it was a bit troubling to see this letter at her bedside. She had an incident yesterday in which intervention with the ambu bag was necessary.

It is interesting to learn that the finance department has had several conversations with me concerning an acceptable payment. I specifically asked about arranging a payment plan but there was no response to that request. I recall receiving a bill for services that were not being provided to my mother.

If I had not addressed the issue of inaccurate charges, my mother would have been charged $36,000.00 more than the actual bill. She was being charged for vent and therapy services that were no longer being provided.

I am interested in having a payment plan as I will not be able to pay $24,000.00 in one payment. As previously requested, I would like clinical documentation to be sent to Lory Alden. Documentation clearly states that she is not safe to be discharged to home at this time, given mucus plugs and requiring hospitalization.

I realize that it is my responsibility to stay abreast of all that relate to my mom. I try to protect her the best way I can. It was an allergic reaction that brought us to this point. She is allergic to heparin, ARBs, ace inhibitors, fentanyl, Percocet, iodine, and sulfur. As I accompanied her with a nurse from Alexandria rehab to the ENT's appointment, when asked about allergies, the nurse stated, 'no known allergies'. In addition, I received a call from the pre-surgical nurse at the Fairfax hospital who stated that she was told by the nurse at Alexandria rehab that my mother has a feeding tube that is being flushed every shift. The feeding tube was discontinued on 11/13/17. I trust that every patient is getting the care that is needed to ensure safety.

Thank you for your time. I look forward to working

with you for a safe discharge plan from Alexandria rehab.

She had requested on at least two occasions that the social worker send her mother's information to the other facility. Since the facility was making it obvious that they were not interested in her mother's safety, she would make every effort to get her out of their care. She also hoped to have her mother closer to her home.

***

On December 14, 2017, Mara received an email from admissions at Lory Alden:

Good evening Mara,

I have received the Application for Admission and POA from you.

I have not received any medical records at all, and receipt of clinical information both from the nursing center in VA as well as her current hospital are needed for us to review for clinical appropriateness for admission. I will not be able to comment on whether or not we will be able to assist/admit her until we have these records to review.

If we can care for her clinically, we will need to discuss her financial situation as well.

Please have both facilities where she has received and is currently receiving care either scan and email to me or fax to 301-000-0000 so we can review.

Thank you.

Were these facilities communicating with each other and passing on negative information? The Alexandria facility wanted Mara to have her mother's house listed for sale for them to be paid fully. They also wanted Mara to apply for Medicaid on her mother's behalf. Mara discussed the Medicaid aspect with her mother who understood that was necessary. The challenge with applying for Medicaid was that Mara did not have all the documents needed for the application and it took some time to collect all the documentation. In the meantime, she did offer to make payments. She concluded that it would have to be greed and perhaps a deliberate wish to be obstructive that would not allow the Alexandria facility to accept a partial payment—but why?

On December 18, 2017, Mara sent another letter to the facility's administrator. It read:

Good morning Mrs. Diane,

I hope this email reaches you well.

I am grateful that my mother has been able to be

weaned off the ventilator at Alexandria rehab. It has been a year that I have been advocating for her trying to get her back home safely. I am requesting that you please assist me in my efforts as this has been exhausting on all accounts for both her and I.

I am prepared to make a payment today of $5,000.00. I would appreciate it if you would accept it as I am interested in making payments on my mother's behalf. Please kindly advise on how I can proceed with this payment. Thank you.

Feeling desperate and wanting to cover all bases, Mara also wrote to the insurance case manager Tori. It was worth a try:

I am writing on my mother's behalf, Denise Mitchell. I appreciate the coverage that the insurance company has allowed thus far, which has allowed her to recover to this point and to be able to participate during her care.
I am asking that the insurance please provide pre-certification for admission to Lory Alden.
She was admitted to Alexandria hospital from 11/20 to 11/24 for respiratory distress after having a mucus plug. I am making the request with the idea that that admission can be considered a new event. There is supporting documentation from two separate ENTs that state that my mother needs to continue skilled nursing care to facilitate safe plugging trials while she works for decannulation. One of the ENTs documented that he is concerned

about the small tube size and that there is a risk of mucus plugging. He recommended that 'she must stay in a setting where she can be monitored' while she still has it.

My mom is not a long-term care candidate. She walks with me once a day, every day when I visit her. Apart from that, she is transferred from the bed to the chair. I was hoping that you would have record of this. I will continue to ask that the staff document when she has walked. I am concerned about complications that could arise due to immobility. She already has had blood clots and pneumonia.

Thank you so much for your time. I am really hoping that the insurance company will afford her the opportunity to improve and to be able to discharge to home soon.

One day passed. Mara received no response from the Alexandria facility. She was becoming anxious. She was contacted by the liaison from the facility on a work-related matter and mentioned that she had not received a response from the Alexandria rehab with regards to her personal letter. That same day, Mara got a response from the facility's administrator, Diane:

Mara,

Our intention of the collections process is never to make someone feel that we are bullying them. We want to work with the resident and the family to ensure that proper payment is made either privately or through an insurance company. We know and understand how difficult it is for residents to understand when they have an outstanding balance, and usually matters are resolved with the Resident Representative. Although seemingly insensitive on the surface to deliver this letter to the resident, it is required by regulation to ensure that they are aware. The letter is delivered with compassion by the accounting department so that any questions can be answered along with the Social Worker so that the resident's psychosocial well-being can be addressed. We never want to cause distress to a resident because the knowledge itself that their bill is outstanding is already very distressful.

Regarding any clinical concerns, I would be happy to meet with you and the nursing team separately to address these.

We look forward to resolving this issue with you. Please let me know (unless one has been sent) a date and time that you can meet with us next week to review her financial situation and what we can do to bring resolution to it for Ms. Mitchell.

Regards,

The issue that Mara had with their process was that her mother had no ability to pay the sum of money that they were asking for. In Mara's estimation, the moment her stay at the facility was no longer covered by the health insurance company, the substandard care that they had already been providing to her, dropped to an even lower level. Mara was terribly upset because she felt that regulations were only applicable to the billing process. Decent quality care and honest, accurate documentation, she felt had nothing to do with regulations.

Diane also indicated that the social worker participated in that compassionate process. Why would Mara want the social worker, who was the same individual who had suggested that Mara list her mother's house, to speak to her mother? It was also the same person whom Mara had asked to send her mother's clinical documentation to another facility. She had had to be reminded several times.

To Diane's suggestion that they have a meeting to discuss the content of Mara's letter, Mara agreed. Mara explained to Diane that she would not be able to attend the meeting in person but that she was available by phone. Diane agreed and further commented that she would have Denise be present at the meeting as well. Mara responded to Diane that her mother should not be present at the meeting for what Mara thought were obvious reasons.

The facility continued to document that Denise had anxiety. She had recently experienced an event that required intervention with the ambu bag; it made no sense to create additional stress for her, Mara thought. Plus, she was not responsible for herself while she was at the rehab, so hearing that they wanted to advertise her house for sale would in no way be helpful to her. Mara had a conversation with her mother and they both agreed that her mother would not be present at the meeting and that Mara would speak on her behalf. Mara also obtained permission from her mother because her friend, Shane, had also offered to participate in the meeting via phone conference to provide support and advice in this grueling experience.

On December 19, 2017, in her efforts to continue to pursue a safe discharge plan from the Alexandria facility for her mother, Mara wrote to admissions at Lory Alden again. She wrote:

Hi Sara,

I am following up with you on the application. I was told by Toni, the insurance case manager (a few days ago) that a request for authorization should be sent from you once you have clinicals from Alexandria rehab. Please keep me updated.

Thanks.

On December 20, 2017, Mara received a response from Lory Alden's admission the next day.

Good afternoon, Mara.

Thank you for your patience in awaiting my reply to your email and voice message. We do not have any available beds at this time for your mother on our Medical Specialty Unit, and do not anticipate having one in the near future.

If/when a bed on our Medical Specialty Unit becomes available, we will consider your mother for admission only after she has been approved by our Medicaid Specialist. The following items will need to be addressed so that if and when a bed opens we will be prepared to give our full attention to her clinical care needs, and have our concerns regarding insurance reimbursement and payment for services settled in advance.

At some point in time, your mother's insurance coverage will come to an end, and she will revert to a Private Pay status. There are important questions that need to be answered before we are able to make a decision regarding our ability to accept your mother to our community. All of her financial information, including her income, assets, outstanding financial obligations and bank statements for the past five years would need to be submitted and reviewed. If you are willing to undergo this process on behalf of your mother, please advise.

Thank you.

Chapter 48

Let's discuss the bill

It was the same day that the meeting was scheduled with the Alexandria rehab. Mara received a phone call from Diane the administrator, as scheduled. Diane started the conversation saying, "so we have your mom here."

Mara responded, "She is not participating in this meeting."

"I spoke with her twice yesterday and she agreed," Diane said. Mara wondered why Diane felt that she had to speak with Denise twice for her to agree. What would have been her motive for having the same conversation twice?

Mara continued, "Well, she must have changed her mind. The last that I knew was that she was not attending this meeting."

454

Diane told Mara that she would talk to Denise. She then moved away from the phone, to do so. After a few minutes, she came back to the phone and said that Denise said, "Mara is handling everything." Diane told Mara, "I just had someone take your mom back to her room." Mara then conferenced her friend Shane to the call.

The meeting began with Diane introducing the participants Edna the unit manager, Carlton the director of respiratory services, Trina the billing specialist, Jolly the social worker and Kari the accounting specialist. Everyone except Kari, Mara and Shane were present in the room. Kari was at another location and was participating via phone conference. The team had intended to have Denise sit alone in the room amongst them, while they intimidated her, was her daughter's belief. Mara was upset. She did not like all that was happening in her mother's care. She felt that they knew that Mara would not be present, so they had planned to make her mother as uncomfortable as possible. It seemed, thought Mara, that presenting Denise with a discharge notice was only a part of the bullying that they had planned. The claim that her mother had anxiety, Mara thought, was only used when they thought it benefited them.

"So, we'll discuss the clinical issues first and then the invoice would be discussed," Diane explained. "You know, we keep those separately."

Mara listened quietly and then stated, "While my mother remains at this facility, my concern is that she gets appropriate care. I want to be sure that the staff caring for her is competent." Diane interrupted, "Really."

Mara continued, "Yes. As I mentioned in the letter, I want to make sure that everyone who is taking care of my mother, is aware of her allergies. Just in case they were missed. My mom is allergic to heparin, ARBs, ACE inhibitors, iodine, Percocet, sulfur, and fentanyl."

Diane stated, "Yes, I see the allergies, but fentanyl is new to the list. How do you know that your mom is allergic to fentanyl?" Mara found Diane to be out of order to question how she Mara, knew that her mother was allergic to fentanyl. She refused to answer that question because she felt that she did not owe any explanation to Diane or anyone else about her knowledge of her mother's allergies.

She considered the fact that Diane, a registered nurse, knew that Mara was also a registered nurse. In Mara's mind, if Diane had a mother whom she cared about and who had experienced what Denise had experienced with an allergic reaction to a medication, she would be interested in preventing another life-threatening event or in the case of fentanyl, for her to be drowsy for days.

"My mom is not to receive fentanyl." She continued, "As a matter of fact, the same nurse who commented at the ENT's office that my mother does not have any allergies was the one who reported to the presurgical nurse at the hospital, that there is a feeding tube that is being flushed. I am mentioning all these issues because they're real and since we all want my mother to be safe, those are some of the issues that have been occurring in regard to her care."

There was silence for a moment and then Diane said, "We'll make sure that the chart is updated."

"What about information that is being reported to outside entities that she has a feeding tube and making sure that the nurses are not just reporting old information?" Mara responded.

"I'll look into it," Diane replied.

As Mara continued to address the clinical issues that she thought were important she mentioned, "My mom walks with me daily in the dining room and I was hoping that it would be documented. The nurses see us walking and they even compliment her, so I was hoping that they would document how well she is doing. That would help with placing her at another facility with insurance coverage."

In response to her comments, Edna the unit manager stated, "What I know is that your mom fell when you were transferring her."

Mara was surprised by the response to her comments. "What happened was that we were waiting for a long time to get assistance to get her back to the bed and she could not wait any longer. I assisted her and did not realize that she was not wearing nonskid socks and she slipped. I helped her to the floor."

Edna remarked "It's still a fall." Mara did not continue the conversation with Edna. What seemed clear to her was that the facility thought of all this interaction in antagonistic terms. They were not interested in the patient.

"Well as you know we've been trying to wean your mom off the trach," Carlton said. "We tried again but she could not tolerate it. She lasted a few more minutes than she did previously with the plugging. We will keep trying."

Mara listened and did not have anything to add or ask of Carlton. She was pleased that he did not use the opportunity to blame her for anything associated with her mother's care. Within a minute of the end of Carlton's sentence, Diane said, "Okay, I will ask the clinical folks, respiratory and nursing to leave the room while the accounting part is being discussed."

Mara listened. *Should she care whether they remained in the room? Would the type of care that her mother received have been any different if they heard the specifics of the accounting?* She tried to imagine her mother being in the room for any part of the discussion, what had already passed and what was yet to come. She knew from conversations with her mother that Denise missed being at home but for a second, as her mind wandered off, she wondered if her mother ever thought about her stay at the Alexandria hospital and at Simion hospital. Perhaps—because as she compared them, Mara realized that none had been as unbearable as her stay at the Alexandria rehab. You had to go through these facilities to be able to compare.

Trina's and Kari's focus was on the balance owed to the facility. It was Kari who initiated the discussion, "We have an outstanding balance of almost $24,000.00. We sent you the invoice a few times."

"Yes, I received it," Mara responded. "I stated that I would be interested in having a payment plan and before I had the opportunity there was a discharge notice."

"We've been waiting for documents for the Medicaid application," Trina responded.

Shane followed with, "I think we all want to have this behind us, right. This has been a lot for

Mara as she has been dealing with her mom at the facility. She has a lot that she has taken on all by herself. Can you tell us what specifically you are waiting for Mara to provide you with?"

In response to the question, Trina remarked, "We need your mom's paystubs and bank statements."

Mara replied, "I am working toward obtaining all the documents that you are requesting but I do not have immediate access to all my mother's information. She was independent before this all happened and was working. I have to get the documents from her employer, but they have their own process to allow me to access her information. I have gotten some of what is needed like the bank statements, but I do need more time to obtain the paystubs."

She listened for a moment and when there was no response she continued, "I can make payments on behalf of my mom but cannot afford the entire balance. I'll also get the documents needed to provide to the Medicaid specialist."

Mara was relieved that her mother was not present at the meeting. She believed that her mother would have been stressed especially at the thought that she had an outstanding balance at the facility that she could not afford and for which she was being evicted. There was static on the phone and after a few minutes, they all got disconnected from the call. About two minutes after the call dropped, the social worker, Jolly, called Mara.

"I am sorry we are having connection problems. They are working on the phone lines. I will email an update."

About five minutes later, Mara received an email from Jolly:

Hello,

Our phone system will be off and on for the next 20 mins, Trina will be giving you a call Mara when the testing is completed.

Thanks

As Jolly had indicated, ten minutes later, Mara received a call from Trina who stated, "I think we were basically finished. You can get the documents to the Medicaid specialist, and he will work on it."

Feeling emotionally and mentally drained from the experience, Mara replied, "Okay. Thanks." They ended the call.

She was sad and wanted to do everything that she could. She wanted the facility to acknowledge the payment offer and not have her mother be the subject of what she thought was harassment. What did it mean that they had not said anything about her offer of a $5000 payment?

Before leaving work that afternoon, Mara received a phone call from Sara at Lory Alden. Sara said to Mara, "Tell me about the discharge notice that you've received from the Alexandria rehab."

Mara was surprised by the question because it seemed to have taken a while before Jolly from the Alexandria facility was able to send clinical information to Lory Alden. When Jolly finally sent the information, she included the discharge notice for nonpayment.

Mara explained, "My mother is now private pay at the Alexandria rehab, but I have spoken with the insurance company, and I was led to believe that she will be covered with new authorization."

Mara knew that it was better to be honest and would not try to deceive any facility. She wanted her mother to get the best care.

"Well. We do not have any beds right now," Sara replied. "I can't promise when one will become available."

"Thanks Sara. I will remain optimistic."

***

Later that evening, Mara entered her mother's room. Denise was sitting upright in the bed. She smiled when she saw her daughter. Mara gave her mother a hug and then said, "What happened today? I thought you were not going to attend the meeting?"

"Somebody came and brought me to the dining room," Denise replied. "They did not say where I was going. I thought you were coming that is why they were taking me there."

Mara looked at her mother questioningly. She said, "Somebody?" Her mother nodded and said, "Yes."

Mara was too annoyed to even bother to ask who took her mother to the dining room. She did not think that it mattered at that point. Denise was accustomed to being taken out of the room, to sit in front of the nursing station while she waited for Mara. It was understandable to Mara if her mother had assumed that she, Mara, was on the way.

They changed the subject and began to talk about Mara's day at work. Denise always wanted to be updated and her daughter enjoyed filling her mother in on the events of her day. They exercised a little and continued to watch television for the rest of the evening until visiting hours ended.

Chapter 49

Persevering to safer ground

On December 21, 2017, Mara was not giving up on working towards getting her mother placed elsewhere. The skilled nursing facility was walking distance from Denise's home. Alstry was one that Mara considered for a while; however, they did not normally accept patients with new tracheostomies. Mara was hopeful for an exception. She spoke with the admission's liaison for Alstry, Abigail, and was optimistic about a transfer.

"My mom has a balance at the Alexandria facility," She informed Abigail. "They gave her a discharge notice for nonpayment, and they sent that notice to Lory Alden who then said that they did not know when a bed would become available."

"Wow. They did that?" Abigail responded. Mara continued, "I'm requesting that the insurance company would consider providing authorization for a transfer to Alstry, given my mother's latest admission to the hospital. Abigail, she is not long-term care. I am planning to have her come home after rehab and hopefully without a trach."

Mara trusted the liaison as they had a good working relationship. Her mother had asked her about that facility for some time. Denise was excited to mouth the words to her sister Simone when she visited her from Grenada, "I can walk home from Alstry."

Mara was incredibly pleased to see her mother excited about any possibility of leaving the Alexandria facility and being so close to her house. It was nice to see her speak with enthusiasm and to have something to look forward to. Mara did not consider it to be false hope because she still believed that everything was possible and that nothing lasted forever. Her aim was to get her mother under the care of competent and compassionate providers. She needed to be on safer ground. She requested that Jolly send her mother's clinical documentation to Alstry.

Mara and Elisa, the healthcare advocate, continued to communicate about Denise's care and their desire to have her transfer to another facility. Mara received a note from Elisa:

Dear Mara,

I have been meaning to tell you that I spoke at length with Toni this week. She recommends that the home of your choice, so now it may be Alstry, needs to receive the reports and request coverage for admission or pre-certification. She also suggested that Alexandria rehab resubmit for coverage of current services that require skilled nursing and respiratory care. Once this submission is received by the insurance company, the Medical Director will be kept updated for a decision.

For now, the insurance company is in 'waiting mode' so action by providers in request for payment and admission is needed.

I like the idea of your mom being close to home.

I am working from home today.

Warmly

Elisa

Mara sent another follow up to Jolly at the Alexandria rehab in response to acknowledgement of a previous email she had sent:

Thanks Jolly. I am working on getting things resolved with Alexandria rehab. I am also trying to get mom closer to home. Alstry is awaiting the clinicals please.

Mara

In her desperate attempts at ensuring safety for her mother, Mara sent another email to the insurance case manager:

Hi Toni,

I have asked Alexandria rehab to send clinicals to Alstry as Lory Alden has no beds.
I am concerned that my mother is not getting the level of care she needs at Alexandria rehab and that the documentation is not reflective of her true status. I had to point out to billing that she is no longer on the vent. I have also had to correct the pre-surgical nurse at the Fairfax hospital (when my mom was going for surgery) as she had received report from Alexandria rehab that my mom has a feeding tube that's being flushed every shift. That feeding tube was discontinued on 11/13/17.
Please advise as to how I may assist to get my mom where she needs to be.

Thank you so much.

The next day, December 22, 2017, Mara followed up with the liaison from Alstry. Abigail said, "They are considering your mom but with the new trach and all, it is a decision that has to be made by the director of nursing. I will give you an answer next week."

It was already Friday afternoon. Mara replied, "Okay Abigail. I am being hopeful. We really need this. Fingers crossed." Mara had not received a response from Toni regarding authorization. She did not make assumptions about the lack of response from Toni as there could be several reasons why she had not responded. If the insurance had planned to provide authorization, they would communicate that information directly to the receiving facility and not necessarily to the family, she concluded. It was also likely that Jolly had not sent any clinical documentation to Alstry because as Mara had experienced with her in the past, nothing regarding Denise was urgent.

Night of the phone call

Later that evening after work, Mara made what was by now a routine trip to the facility to visit her mother. It was a Friday evening. The time was six o'clock. As she entered her mother's room, Denise was sitting on the bedside commode and there was a nursing assistant who was attending to her. Denise did not want the assistant to continue to attend to her or she just wanted Mara to attend to her. Denise said, "Mara clean me."

Mara immediately realized that the inner cannula to her mother's tracheostomy needed to be cleaned. The pattern was that her voice was audible whenever she needed to be suctioned and to have the inner cannula for the tracheostomy cleaned. She did not tolerate the passy muir, speaking valve and the audible voice was the indicator that she needed respiratory services. But if she knew that, wouldn't a nursing assistant at the facility know that, too? Did they just not care? Or did they not have the training that, she felt, should be required before they were able to assist patients without supervision? Denise was still sitting on the commode. She was not cleaned.

Mara placed her bag on the chair. Before she could approach her mother, the nursing assistant retorted, "Ms. Mitchell relax."

So, she thought, they are going to read it as anxiety. She said, "It is not anxiety. She is having a respiratory problem."

One of the nurses on the unit, Sania, was passing in the hallway and must have heard Mara's comment. She entered the room and dealt with Denise's trach. Denise was clearly having difficulty breathing. Her chest was rising quickly, and she complained, "My chest feels so tight."

Sania removed the inner cannula. Mara could see that the little device was clogged with mucus. Sania proceeded to suction Denise's trach. The nurse and nursing assistant cleaned her and assisted her to stand. They moved a few steps closer to the bed. Denise sat on the edge of the bed. A few moments later, Denise's assigned nurse Julia entered the room and realized what was happening. She asked Denise, "How do you feel?"

Both nurses stood in front of Denise. As Denise continued to use her accessory muscles and still sounding short of breath, she responded, "A little better." Mara looked on and then said, "She needs to be suctioned frequently. The trach is a smaller size, and she tends to have thick mucus. Also, she cannot tolerate sitting in the hallway for extended periods without humidification."

For a moment, Julia glanced over at Mara with furrowed eyebrows, and then continued to speak to Denise, "If you're having chest pain, we're going to have to transfer you to the hospital."

Knowing that her mother wanted to leave that facility, Mara then said to her mother, "If you leave here, you're not coming back."

Julia said, "Mara!" Mara's response showed her total frustration with the facility. Mucus plugs again, issues with the oxygen tank, issues with humidification, issues, issues, issues at this facility. Sometimes, Denise had difficulty with dried stagnant mucus, and that made it even more difficult for her to breathe. Mara knew that Denise wanted to leave the facility because she realized that they were not providing the care that she needed. So, Mara knew that if her mother left the facility, she would do her utmost to have her moved elsewhere so she wouldn't have to return. Mara asked the nurses, "Please check her pulse ox."

They did, as the machine was next to them. The machine indicated that Denise's pulse oximetry was 84%. They increased the amount of oxygen that she was receiving, and her pulse oximetry increased to 91% then gradually to 94%. Imagine! She had to ask for them to check her mother's oxygen level. Another constant issue. Later she wondered if she should have asked for an EKG to be done or insisted that she be transferred to the hospital immediately.

Denise was lethargic and weaker on the left side. She was leaning more to the left. She was responding appropriately but her eyes seemed weak.

Mara asked, "Did she get any new medications because she seems different?"

Julia responded, "No. She did not."

Denise was sleepy. Mara asked her, "Mummy, how are you feeling?"

Denise looked up at her daughter and said with a faint voice, "I'm okay." Mara, in a typical response when her mother seemed worried, tried to change the subject. She said, "So. What do you want for Christmas?" Her mother responded, "You can buy me a chain." Mara smiled and was pleased that her mother asked for something that she could give her. So, she wants a necklace. She was glad that her mother did not say that she wanted to be home for Christmas. Denise drifted off to sleep. Mara stayed at her mother's bedside. She said prayers, praying on her own this time.

"Lord, we need you. Please bless and protect mummy. Keep her safe in the hands of her caregivers. Lord we are hoping for a miracle for her to be accepted at another facility that can provide proper care to her. We want her to eventually be back at her own home. Please let her have a peaceful night sleep and give her the strength she needs to continue to have a full recovery."

She kissed her mother on the cheek. She walked out to the parking area, got into her car, and turned on the ignition. It was almost 8:40pm on December 22, 2017.

***

Mara got to her home and prepared for bed. It took a while before she fell asleep, but she eventually did. She was asleep when her phone rang at 12:52am on December 23, 2017. It was one of the nurses from the Alexandria facility on the line.

Nurse Celina told her, "Your mom was found to be unresponsive. 911 was called and they are working on her."

Mara sat up in the bed. Her hands started to shake. She needed both hands to hold the phone. She tried to make her voice sound strong as she said with a stutter, "When was the last time that she was seen?"

Celina responded, "At 10pm. Are you coming?"

Mara replied, "Yes. Yes, I am."

Celina got off the phone. Mara continued to hold the phone. Shortly after hanging up, nervous Mara called back the facility for an update on her mother's status and was told by the person who answered, "They are still working with her."

She understood that to mean that the emergency personnel were still performing CPR on her mother. She began to get dressed. A few minutes later, Celina called Mara, "They are taking your mom to the Alexandria hospital."

Mara placed the phone on speaker. She put it down on the bed. She was struggling to put on a sweater. It was inside out. She tried again. She asked, "What about her vital signs? Her pulse ox? Is she responding?"

Celina informed her, "Her pulse ox was 70%. She is unconscious."

Mara was in no condition to drive. Not only was she sleepy but she was also overwhelmed with a multitude of emotions: concerned, worried, afraid, helpless, nervous, and angry. According to the nurse, the emergency personnel worked with her mother for several minutes and even as she left the facility to be transferred to the hospital, she remained unresponsive.

Mara called her Aunt Myrna to let her know about the call from the rehab. Her aunt suggested that she take Uber. The ride to the hospital took an hour. To her, it took much longer this time. She called her friend Shane. He stayed on the phone with her until the Uber arrived at the hospital.

On arrival to the hospital, Mara waited for a couple of hours before she was allowed to see her mother on the critical care unit. She spoke with the intensivist via telephone as she sat in the waiting room. She was told, "Your mom remains unresponsive. We are waiting to do a CT scan of her brain. Her heart rhythm is erratic. She is also having some twitching in her face. There is a lot going on. Her liver is not functioning. She has multiple organ dysfunction."

Mara listened quietly. She was afraid. The intensivist continued, "She has had a few cardiac arrests tonight." Each statement sounded worse than the last. She remained in the waiting room after she spoke with the intensivist. Mara prayed.

"Lord, we really need you. Please let mummy be okay. She has come a long way. We are depending on you to see her pull through this.

Mara wished that the weekend had passed and that she had already received acceptance from Alstry for her mother and authorization from the insurance company. Even though her mother was under the care of health care professionals, she wished that she had thought of everything that needed to be done that evening. She knew there was no guarantee that her suggestions would have been acknowledged, but she could have said something. She wished that she had insisted that her mother needed to be transferred to the hospital immediately to have diagnostic tests and labs drawn. She wondered about the actual amount of time that had passed since anyone had checked on her mother after she left the facility that evening.

On December 23, 2017, Mara sat in the waiting room and continued to pray. After several more minutes, one of the nurses from the critical care unit arrived at the waiting room and escorted her to the unit. Mara entered her mother's room and saw that she was being attended to by several nurses. Her mother was unconscious. She was on full ventilator support. Denise was unable to do anything. The ventilator was breathing for her. They were giving her various blood products:

platelets, plasma, red blood cells. She was in multi-organ failure. Mara had been told the same thing about her mother, when she was at the Northern Metropolitan Hospital. What? Multi-organ failure? This time, though, it was different. Denise was bleeding profusely from every orifice. She had developed what was termed disseminated intravascular coagulation (DIC). This is a condition in which abnormal clumps of thickened blood clots form inside blood vessels. The clots use up the blood's clotting factors, which can then lead to massive bleeding from many sites of the body. As Denise continued to receive more blood products, the bleeding continued. There were two nurses at her side who applied pressure to stop the bleeding. Mara offered to take one of the nurse's place and allowed her to perform other functions for her mother.

Mara talked to her, "Mummy you have come a long way. I am so proud of you. I know you can do this. Just keep fighting and praying. You have done such an excellent job and you have a lot of support. There are a lot of prayer groups that are lifting you up in prayers."

Mara held her mother's hand and told her, "I am right here. I am going to continue to fight for you."

Mara was not ready to let her mother go. She worried about the bleeding but still prayed for a miracle. She knew about DIC but never actually had a patient who was in DIC. The nurses were very supportive. They empathized with Mara. The male nurse who was also applying pressure to Denise's nostril and groin said, "I know this must be difficult. I am sorry."

She held back the tears as much as she could because she did not want the nurses to focus on her. She wanted them to continue to do everything that they could to save her mother's life.

The intensivist led Mara to the consultation room. As they entered the room and sat down, he said, "Your mom is extremely ill. I see that she is full code. Have you thought about changing her status to do not resuscitate? We will continue to treat her but if her heart stops again, do you want us to perform CPR? She has had several cardiac arrests tonight. You can think about it. Talk to your family."

Mara, feeling sad and scared, responded, "No. I cannot change it. She came too far. I cannot change it to do not resuscitate right now. She survived two aortic dissections. The second one was a year ago and it was a reaction from a medication that caused her to be placed back on the ventilator. Then a number of complications followed. She managed to get off the ventilator and just needed to tolerate plugging of the trach. That was the main reason she was still at the rehab."

The intensivist listened and then asked Mara, "When was the last time that you saw your mom?" Mara responded, "Last night. I see her every day at the facility. She got to the point where she was walking with me using a walker. She is alert, oriented to person, place, time, and situation."

He interrupted, "Did she seem normal?" Mara said, "When I arrived yesterday, she was having respiratory issues as I could hear her voice and that is the indication that the trach needed to be suctioned as she was not tolerating the passy muir valve. She also started to complain of chest pain. The nurse told her that they would send her to the hospital if she was having chest pain but after the inner cannula was cleaned and she was suctioned she said that she was feeling better. She started to become sleepy. I stayed for a while longer and left. Then about four hours or so later, I got a call from the facility saying that they found her unresponsive."

The intensivist was kind to Mara. He just listened. She asked him, "Do you think that it is possible that the respiratory distress that she was having could have led to cardiac arrests?"

He responded, "It is possible. Your mom also has sepsis."

Mara explained to him about her observations at the facility, "She is not suctioned frequently enough at the rehab. Her trach was changed from size six to a size four and she has a lot of thick mucus which she has trouble getting through the smaller trach." She paused. Her hands were shaking. She struggled to hold back tears. She tried to reason her way through all this. She continued, " I have had to request many times that she gets suctioned but it seems as though they're allowing stagnant mucus to build up in her lungs. Now, I suppose they have traveled through her blood stream."

Mara recalled at the care plan meeting when she asked Dr. Kulkarti to send cultures from her mother's sputum and from secretions from the tracheostomy but those were not sent to her knowledge.

The intensivist said to Mara, "You hang in there. We will do everything we can for your mom. If you decide to change her code status, have her nurse call me."

He left her in the consultation room while she sat there thinking how different things could have been for her mother. Thinking: it is the health care system. She had lots of issues, but things could have been different. If she had the best care possible, things could be different.

Chapter 50

Peaceful sleep

As daybreak came on December 23, 2017, Mara texted family and friends about her mother's admission to the hospital. It was her Aunt Yvonne's birthday in Grenada. She called her on the phone. Instead of wishing her aunt a happy birthday, she said, "Mummy is in the hospital and things are not looking good."

She could barely get the words out. She began to cry. She received an abundance of responses with support and concern. One of her mother's friends Glory, arrived at the hospital within an hour to bring breakfast for Mara. She kept her company while they waited for her mother's condition to improve. Mara spoke with her mother's friend Ali, a retired physician for medical advice and emotional support.

Her aunt Ali explained more about DIC to Mara. She advised her to be specific in making sure that the staff knows that she is not withdrawing care but simply changing the code status if that was the decision that Mara wanted to make. The staff needed to get a response from Mara as they continued to transfuse more blood products. Her mother's friends, her aunts Breana, Lori, Mena, and Myrna arrived. Aunt Cathy was away but remained in touch. Breana provided support to Mara. She told her "Whatever your decision, it would be the right one and I would support you."

Mara called her brother but was unable to reach him. She heard from her friend Hilda in Grenada who listened to her while she cried on the phone. She spoke with her friend Shane who also provided words of encouragement. She needed to decide on her mother's code status and realized that her mother had lost a significant amount of blood throughout the previous night. It seemed unlikely that her mother would recover from her condition. Mara said to her mother's nurse, "Can I talk to the intensivist?"

The nurse replied, "Sure" and she dialed his number and handed Mara the wireless phone. Mara stood outside of her mother's room, in the doorway.

She told him, "This is an extremely difficult decision for me to make." She paused.

"I understand," he said. "We would continue to provide care to your mom."

Mara continued, "I have decided to have my mother's code status changed to do not resuscitate." Within a minute of conveying her decision to the intensivist, as she walked to her mother's side and held her hand, the overhead monitor flat-lined.

Denise had moved on to be with her heavenly Father. Perhaps she wanted to know that Mara was okay with her leaving her. It was a peaceful goodbye, but it was not one that Mara was ready for. She stood there in shock. She knew what was happening but could not believe that it was happening—that it had happened. Her mother was gone.

Her aunts Lori and Mena were standing outside of the room, but the shock did not allow her to speak to let them know. She could not say anything to them and just assumed that they knew. They realized after hearing the nurse on the phone at the nursing station and entered the room. The other ladies who were present earlier had already left due to their own obligations. Life did not stop in other places while one important part of it moved on.

While at the Alexandria rehab, Denise had been making progress; therefore, no one had been expecting that outcome. They got the news of her death on arrival to the hospital. Mara's phone rang.

She answered, "Hello." On the other end was her mother's friend Maitland.

He said, "Mara, I just went to the rehab to see your mom. They told me she is in the hospital. I left a gift for her."

Tears rolled down Mara's face. She said, "Mr. Maitland, I am sorry, mummy passed."

She heard the gasp in his voice. He said, "What? Oh no. I am so sorry. I will check on you later." They ended the call.

Her mother's colleague Enid arrived. Mara's friends Becka and Mikala arrived separately. Denise's ex-husband Matt, her primary care physician and Denise's son Malcolm also arrived. Mara stood with them on the right side of her mother's bed. Her eyes were red. She was extremely sad. She thought about her mother, bringing people together once again. In the room across from them, Denise lay unmoving.

Epilogue

The delivery of health care at every health care institution must be held at the same high standard. Nursing facilities, whether short-term or long-term care should not be excused for providing suboptimal service. Organizations should not be allowed to resemble health care facilities; they either are, or they are not. There is great urgency for transparency at health care facilities, as can be seen with the COVID-19 pandemic. COVID-19 has placed nursing homes in the spotlight. Not all facilities are inadequate, but where inadequacy is seen there, it is a symptom of something much larger and more corrosive in the health care system generally.

Patients or residents, the vulnerable population at nursing facilities rely on caregivers to keep them safe. Communicable diseases at any nursing facility should be made public. The public has a right to make informed decisions, especially as they try to determine where to place loved ones. The positive cases for COVID-19 should include both staff and residents alike. Some states have decided to publicize the number of COVID cases and deaths at nursing facilities, but not Arizona. As recent as May 20, 2020, the nursing homes in Arizona were not required by law to publicly reveal their number of positive COVID-19 cases. This is a significant issue and must be regarded as such. If nursing homes begin to get passes on critical matters that prove to be deadly especially among the vulnerable population, can this population expect protection in other areas?

How can this transparency be achieved? Look at states such as California, New Jersey and Massachusetts that have prioritized mandatory testing early during the pandemic, of all staff at nursing homes. Reports of positive coronavirus cases have also been made public. While the facilities have done well with restricting visitors, the patients and residents may contract the virus from caregivers at the facilities; therefore, testing all staff is essential for the delivery of safe care. The states have found that reports of coronavirus cases at the nursing facilities have been beneficial in terms of understanding where the problems exist and allow authorities the opportunity to implement measures to address the issues and develop policies.

Are the facilities providing their workers with all the necessary personal protective equipment? It is not sufficient to provide the protective gear, but it is imperative to ensure that the workers are professionally trained to use the protective gear. Are they trained to wash their hands properly? There must be more oversight at the facilities. Infection control measures need to be in place for nursing facilities. This does not only apply to coronavirus, but it speaks to a broader issue of infection. Are the caregivers at the facilities trained to identify symptoms of infection? Patients and residents rely on health care professionals when they seek care at these facilities. Anything less than the care that is needed is not acceptable.

Lack of transparency will only serve the interests of shareholders of the facilities. There will be no benefit to patients. The concern by those in Arizona who are withholding information from the public, is privacy. No one needs to know the individuals' names who have been affected with COVID. A count of the number of cases at each facility will suffice. Allowing potential residents to be misled or to make uninformed decisions only benefits those who have monetary interests in the nursing homes.

Families of patients or residents who are affected by COVID also need to be notified.

Nursing facilities should not be allowed to conceal information that will provide answers to grieving families. Rules must be in place with frequent monitoring to ensure that nursing homes and health care facilities are operating at an acceptable standard. The enforcement of the rules should be accompanied with fines, revoking of accreditation for facilities and loss of licensure for individual staff.

States that have difficulty in governing nursing homes and health care facilities should seek and receive assistance from the federal government. Nursing homes which receive funding from Medicare and Medicaid should be required by these programs to provide a high level of care. These programs should also require transparency to continue to receive funds. If the nursing facilities are held accountable for the care or lack of care that they provide and their funding is affected, they may be inclined to change. Information from patients and patients' families should be an important part of the review procedure for these facilities.

Resources:

* Medicare

- Department of Health and Human Services

- Congressional representative

- Nursing Home Ombudsman

About the Author

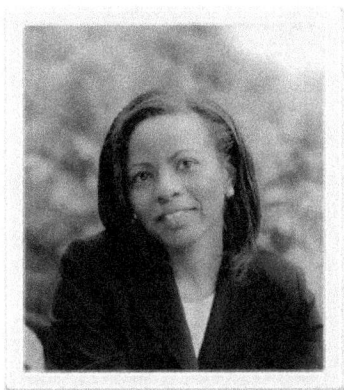

Marilyn Mitchell is a first-time author with more than 20 years of experience in the healthcare industry. Born in the United States and of Caribbean descent, she grew up in Grenada, West Indies. Marilyn has over 15 years as a Registered Nurse and worked in areas such as Women's Surgery, Post-Anesthesia Care Unit and Case Management. She spent 10 years in utilization management and discharge planning. A constant that defines her entire career is her passionate advocacy for patients' rights and humane practices in a healthcare system that too often does not have them as a priority. She holds a Master of Science in Healthcare Administration and Master of Business Administration from the University of Maryland Global Campus (2014); a Bachelor of Science in Nursing from University of Maryland Baltimore (2010); an Associate Degree in Nursing from Montgomery College (2006); and a Bachelor of Science in Health Management from Howard University (1998). She is a certified case manager.

www.ingramcontent.com/pod-product-compliance
Lightning Source LLC
Chambersburg PA
CBHW030233030426
42336CB00009B/79